ADVANCED TECHNOLOGY IN COMMERCE, OFFICES AND HEALTH SERVICES

Advanced Technology in Commerce, Offices and Health Services

Edited by
FE JOSEFINA DY
International Labour Office

A study prepared for the International Labour Office

Avebury

Aldershot · Brookfield USA · Hong Kong · Singapore · Sydney

© International Labour Organisation 1990

Published by
Avebury
Gower Publishing Company Limited
Gower House, Croft Road
Aldershot, Hants GU11 3HR
England

Gower Publishing Company
Old Post Road
Brookfield, Vermont 05036
USA

British Library Cataloguing in Publication Data
Advance technology in commerce, offices and health services
 : a study prepared for the International Labour Office.
1. Work. Orginazation. Implications of technological
innovation
I. Dy, F. J. (Fe Josefina) 1947-   II. International Labour
Office
306.36

ISBN   0-566-07156-8

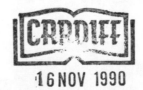

Printed in Great Britain by
Athenaeum Press Ltd, Newcastle upon Tyne.

Table of contents

3. Computer-aided office work: Concepts and research findings

by "Computer-Aided Office Work" Research Group, Work and Organisational Psychology Unit, Swiss Federal Institute of Technology

ILO preface

The International Labour Office has as an essential mission the protection of workers throughout the world. In order to carry out this mission, it co-operates with governments and organisations of employers and workers in the identification of problems and practical solutions. ILO activities in the field of conditions of work have been reinforced through the International Programme for the Improvement of Working Conditions and Environment (PIACT).

New technologies affect the conditions of work of a rapidly increasing number of workers in all sectors. The consequences of introducing these technologies are far-reaching and complex, and appropriate responses are often difficult to identify and implement. In order to explore the concrete implications of new technologies in the specific sectors of commerce, offices and health services, the ILO has called upon noted experts in several countries. They have analysed both national situations and developments in particular work settings. Their studies, together with a comparative introduction, show the diversity of technological developments, the key role of organisational choices and the opportunities and dangers for both management and workers.

1 Introduction

F. J. DY

Today there is enormous interest about the effects of new technology on workers in commerce, offices and health services. This is clear from the numerous conferences, studies, policies and programmes dealing with this topic. New regulations, collective agreements, guide-lines, model codes and training programmes concerning the introduction of technology proliferate.

This interest is not difficult to explain. In most advanced countries, the majority of workers are white-collar workers. The service sector has grown at the expense of manufacturing and agriculture. Service sector growth has been accompanied by a rapid increase in the number and proportion of women in the labour force. In what Daniel Bell has called the "information society", the handling of facts and figures, data and text has become the most labour-intensive activity. Numerous studies have tried to calculate the number of "information-related jobs" – that is, jobs primarily related to the processing of information. The OECD placed the figure, depending on the country concerned, between 27 and 41 per cent of the labour force in the mid-1970s. But because such jobs are difficult to classify, these are rough estimates. There can be no doubt, however, that access to information and decision-making rather than machine power and physical labour are the dominant factors in the emerging post-industrial economy.

Competition within the service sector is also becoming more intense as new technology breaks down many of the boundaries between industries. For example, banks, insurance companies and brokerage houses increasingly offer a similar range of services and compete head-to-head on the basis of location, knowledge and cost. Even retail

1

stores and manufacturing companies have used their strengths in consumer credit to offer similar financial service packages. Services have also restructured the national and international marketplace. Communication technologies permit manufacturers to co-ordinate design, distribution and marketing strategies on a nation-wide or world-wide basis. Thus services have become a critical cost dimension in marketing and manufacturing competitiveness.

New technology will continue to be widely introduced, and will affect a significant proportion of workers in offices, commerce and health services. Increased demands for information processing and the need to increase productivity and reduce costs will continue to be important reasons for its introduction. Today, the question is no longer whether organisations will introduce new technology, but when and how they will do it.

The growth of work using new technology has posed questions about its consequences – how it affects jobs and skill requirements, organisational structures, working conditions and the performance of individuals and organisations. These questions about consequences, of course, are directly related to questions about choices and policies during the planning and introduction of technology; implicitly they concern the organisational goals, politics and economic interests that underlie such choices.[1] Since new technologies are extremely flexible and versatile, organisations may select, adapt and use them in almost unlimited ways. The consequences, therefore, reflect organisational planning and the management of change strategies.

This study is part of an ongoing ILO programme of research on the implications of new technology for the quality of working life. It builds on and supplements other projects which have resulted in the publication of *Automation and work design* by F. Butera and J.E. Thurman (Amsterdam, North Holland, 1984), *Visual display units: Job content and stress in office work* by F.J. Dy (Geneva, ILO, 1985) and the *Conditions of Work Digest*, "Special issue on visual display units" (Geneva, ILO, 1986).

This study brings together the work of researchers from the Federal Republic of Germany, Hungary, Japan, Norway, Switzerland and the United Kingdom. These researchers were already carrying out studies on new technology and work organisation in offices and the service sector. They were requested to adapt, to the extent possible, their current or previous work to a common research design. Financial constraints did not allow the commissioning of new studies by the ILO.

The objectives of the study are to describe the main technologies which are being used in offices, commerce and health services, together with their implications for organisational structure and job characteristics, and to explore issues related to technological and organisational choices and the future of work in the service sector. It is important to point out that while the effects of new technology on employment have become major social issues, they are not the focus of this study. Some country reports, however, have included a discussion of these issues as part of the background for the changes occurring in the nature or quality of jobs and the working life of workers.

The country reports vary in how they describe the impact of technology on workers. This is perhaps a reflection of the complexity of the issues being examined and of the importance of wider social, political and economic factors. Methodologically, different approaches were used: questionnaires, individual interviews, group interviews, analyses of various surveys and studies, and so on. In several instances, a "before-and-after" approach was used in the case studies.

In spite of the different technologies and the varied organisational settings covered, the national reports illustrate some common themes and come to quite similar conclusions. These themes and conclusions relate to the positive and negative implications of technological change for organisational structure, jobs and organisational choice.

In this introduction, the types of technology commonly applied in offices, commerce and health services are described first because technology is often considered a major driving force in organisational change. Moreover, because offices, stores and hospitals are parts of complex organisations, one can look at the impact of new technology at several levels. Thus, the second part of the introduction examines some of the implications of technological change for organisational structure. The organisation as a whole may be affected: its decision-making may become more or less centralised, its size may decrease, its geographical location may be altered and its interactions with customers, suppliers and competitors may change. However, the most commonly discussed impacts of new technology usually focus on people. The effects of new technology on jobs is the third theme covered in this introduction. For example, individual-oriented issues, such as responsibility and autonomy on the job, career prospects, skills and qualifications and communication patterns, are often used as criteria on which the effects of new technologies are assessed. In many ways, these effects reflect the values and choices of decision-makers. The final theme, technological and organisational choice, is ultimately what the study is about. Organisational choice is *the* issue. This is clear from the country reports: the same technology in similar organisational settings but with different organisational choices produces different effects.

3

Technology

The country reports describe the general-purpose technologies commonly used in offices, supermarkets and retail stores, and in computerised laboratories and intensive care in hospitals. They range from simple keypunch machines and electronic cash registers to complex on-line systems and advanced networks.

While the rates of development and diffusion of computer-based technology vary between the countries and industries studied, they seem to follow a similar pattern. Computerisation of office work has undergone two phases: a period of centralised computing and a period of integrated and decentralised microelectronic-based technology. In the first phase, electronic data processing (EDP) was used for highly structured routine administrative procedures, such as payroll processing, invoicing, bookkeeping, and certain kinds of typing. Computer functions tended to be centralised in certain departments or in EDP centres. Processing took place off-line in "batch runs", often requiring extensive manual preparation. The second phase began with the application of microelectronic-based technology. The increased computing and storage capacity of the new technology facilitated the decentralisation of information processing. So-called "intelligent" terminals allowed data to be processed locally and to be transmitted efficiently to geographically dispersed units and departments. Software packages allowed people with a limited knowledge of computers or programming to manipulate text and quantitative data, to generate tables and graphic displays, and to exchange information with other computer users without the intervention of computer specialists. On-line or real-time systems gradually replaced off-line systems or the batch processing of data.

In some countries (e.g. Japan) and in some industries (e.g. banking), the third phase of computerisation has already begun. Microcomputers are linked to other microcomputers, mainframe computers or minicomputers and such linked systems are also connected with outside communication systems to create "integrated office systems". Networking will become increasingly a major trend in the computerisation of office work.

The most widely discussed type of new office technology is the word processor. It has already replaced the typewriter in many offices. Word processors vary considerably in sophistication, in their capacity to handle large volumes of work and in the range of special features they offer. However, they all consist basically of five components: a keyboard (similar to the keyboard of a conventional typewriter but with additional command keys); a visual display screen (for displaying text typed or retrieved from

4

memory); a central processing unit (the power source and computing part of the word processor); a storage unit or memory (it may be in the form of floppy or hard disks, magnetic card or cassette); and a printer.

The introduction of new technology has been more widespread in banking and financial services than in any of the other service industries. Many banks have introduced integrated systems of computers, telecommunication and electronic equipment. Terminals have been introduced for processing cheques and credit, for enquiries from customers and for the production of reports. Counter terminals which capture data as transactions take place are also used. In addition, many banks have introduced automatic teller machines (ATMs) which dispense cash and answer routine enquiries such as account balances or requests for statements and chequebooks. Payment by electronic funds transfer (EFT) is increasingly becoming common.

New technology in commerce and retailing is often associated with electronic point-of-sale (POS) terminals. POS is the general name given to electronic cash registers which collect information at the cash desk or check-out counter. POS was first introduced in the United States in the early 1970s as a means of integrating buying operations with sales in such a way as to reduce stockholding. By laser scanning, keying-in coded data or using a magnetic wand, itemised commodities could be monitored and controlled across sales outlets, however geographically remote. As noted in the report on the United Kingdom, the greatest promise for POS was the possibility of an integrated retailing system. With the automatic reordering of goods on the basis of current sales and stocks (purchase order management), the system allows the automatic refurbishing of stockrooms from company warehouses and deliveries from producers, wholesalers or manufacturers without the human processing of orders. While this system is prevalent in the United States, it is still more or less experimental in many European countries where sales information is more often used as a guide by buyers in head offices and by local managers.

One of the major reasons for the slow development and diffusion of advanced technology in commerce in comparison with other branches of the service sector was the length of time taken by European manufacturers to agree to and to adopt a European Article Numbering System (EAN).

In the health sector, the technology described in the reports includes computerised analytical equipment (Hungary and the United Kingdom) and microelectronic-based patient monitoring in intensive care units (United Kingdom). Auto-analysers are now used in most biochemistry laboratories to test samples of blood, urine and other body fluids.

5

Previously, this was done by mixing samples with appropriate chemicals and physically shaking them or submitting them to centrifugal force in order to separate them into analysable forms. Test results were often printed out in graphs which were interpreted and calculated by technicians. Today, auto-analysers provide a complete profile of one or several specimens which have been submitted to a battery of tests; the results are transmitted "on-line" to a computer which prints them out or displays them on a screen.

The introduction of microcomputers has made it possible for readings of vital functions (heart rate, pulse rate, blood pressure and central venous pressures) to be recorded, analysed and displayed on a video monitor in a more sophisticated way than is possible using pen and paper. In some intensive care units, monitors may be connected to central nursing stations or on-line to computers handling data on patients. Although still relatively rare, computerised data-information systems for patients have been introduced in the United Kingdom. Interconnected terminals and video screens are placed at the bedsides of patients, in laboratories and in operating rooms.

There is little doubt that new technologies can be powerful tools at work. Unlike "automation", which is commonly understood as computer-controlled execution of highly structured routines, microelectronics-based technology can be used to support and augment work that is variable, heterogeneous and complex.

Discussions and decision-making still tend to focus on hardware, which represents a relatively small part of the total system cost and is getting cheaper all the time. Questions on technology tend to become a proxy for addressing more difficult and perhaps more controversial problems and issues concerning organisational and work design, worker attitudes and management-worker relationships.

Implications for organisational structure

The structural changes described in the country reports cover a wide range. They include, for example, the establishment of centralised labelling and purchasing departments in commerce (Federal Republic of Germany, Japan and the United Kingdom), the emergence of a "new professional type of hierarchy which exercises control over activities affected by the new technology" (Hungary), the establishment of local word processing centres to service several bank branches (Japan) and the establishment of an integrated customer service in banks, which combines functions relating to customer accounts, credit and investments that were

6

previously in separate departments (Federal Republic of Germany, Japan and the United Kingdom).

The reports illustrate the three most common types of structural change – the integration of departments, greater functional specialisation and reduction in the number of hierarchical levels – which occur when new technology is introduced in bureaucratic organisations.

Since the technology allows the integration of information from many sources and the distribution of information to many locations, departments whose activities can be incorporated into a computer information system are often integrated. For example, with the establishment of an integrated customer service system in banks, separate departments no longer handle customer accounts, credit and loans, investments and foreign transactions. Similarly, the creation of EDP departments in banks has resulted in the absorption of departments concerned with bookkeeping and other records. Such integration of departments is especially likely if there is a reduction in staff.

The introduction of new technology can also lead to the creation of new departments with functional specialities. Previously, departments were often structured so that they dealt with all or most of the activities related to a particular product or geographical area. Today, in spite of other options, there is a tendency to follow the logic of computer systems and to create departments, such as centralised word-processing pools and data preparation departments, centralised pricing and purchasing departments and specialised query departments. This development, which is in many ways the opposite of the first, is especially likely in companies with many branches which see opportunities for economies of scale through carrying out some activities on a company-wide basis. At the same time, work within the functional departments has tended to become polarised into "expert" and "routine" tasks. The report of the Federal Republic of Germany notes that the widespread use of EDP in offices has often led to a new division of labour where "subsidiary employees do the collection of data, preliminary sorting of information, archiving, documentation and winding-up procedures and experts process the aspects of procedures (e.g. negotiations, qualitative assessment of applications) which are relevant to decision-making".

A reduction in the number of levels in the hierarchy often occurs, especially when fewer people are employed. Integration or functional arrangement of departments can also result in fewer hierarchical levels. This is particularly obvious when the computer takes over many of the control and checking functions, which were previously done by people in a specific level of the hierarchy. For example, as is seen in the case studies of British and Japanese banking, the functions of controlling the work, balancing, and checking transactions are now largely carried out by the computer. The banks have adopted broadly a two-tier structure of cashiers on the counter and senior managerial staff who deal with loans, investments and specialised banking. This polarisation of abilities and work content has significant implications for flexibility and variety of work within banks and the career opportunities for junior staff.

These developments are related to another effect which is often associated with the introduction of new technology: increased centralised control within and between organisations. The capacity of computer systems, especially on-line systems, to process enormous amounts of information quickly and easily facilitates their use in regulating and co-ordinating the activities of departments. For example, the Japanese report describes a 1983 survey carried out by the Ministry of International Trade and Industry (MITI) which showed that 40 to 60 per cent of the firms surveyed considered that control by head offices had increased significantly. Such control was evident in that (1) the objectives given to the branches by head offices had become more detailed; (2) the frequency of checking activities by head offices had increased; (3) the directives addressed to branches had become more frequent; and (4) the data or information to be sent to head offices by the branches had increased. Similarly, the British report notes that "sales managers may lose their information gathering and processing function by the new ability at the centre of the company to obtain and analyse data over a much wider area of the companys operation, and with the statistically modelled expertise contained in the information technology". For example, price-item schedules are now obtained from a regional computer unit and hence the departmental manager has lost the authority to alter prices or to organise special sales or promotions.

In Hungary, the possibility of increased centralisation of control was recognised by top managers but they did not consider it their task "to control day-to-day processes at lower levels". However, a tendency toward increased formalisation was noted as procedures were specified and adapted to the functions of the entire information-processing network.

Centralisation of control may often be facilitated by the use of a management information system which allows for the integration of widely differing kinds of information. As noted in the report of the Federal Republic of Germany, programmes are increasingly used for the qualitative assessment of current business activities as well as for planning future business policies and strategies.

In other cases, organisational changes cannot be attributed only or primarily to the introduction of new technology. Enterprises have also made organisational changes as part of a process of rationalisation or "streamlining" to improve efficiency and competitiveness. Although rationalisation may facilitate or precede the introduction of new technology, it is also carried out independently of technological changes. For example, in a "superstore" chain in Japan, decision-making was centralised before the introduction of POS terminals and the computerised system which was introduced eventually supported the centralised decision-making structure. The authors of the British report observed "conditions of increased contest for resources and rationalisation of expenditure accompanied by a growing attempt to assert central standards of control and discipline at the point of service" in the banking, health and retailing industries. They added that "we might indeed be witnessing a trend towards the industrialisation of service work in which technology is playing no more than an enabling role".

Some of the reports (Finland, Hungary, Japan, Norway, Switzerland) offer a different perspective. They point out that while the introduction of new technology can be accompanied by a planned change in work organisation, in many cases what actually happens is the allocation of equipment within the existing organisational structure. New technology is introduced to meet certain efficiency or productivity requirements but to the extent possible without changing the organisational setting. This is exemplified by the two Swiss case studies of planned change in the secretariats of a federal agency and in the central personnel division of a multinational enterprise based in Switzerland. In the first project, aimed at "designing work adapted to human needs", changes were initiated only *within* a particular section or department; any changes *among* departments were excluded. In the second project, the authors were asked to look at the company's plans to modernise its personnel information system "to improve organisational structure using a participative design model". Since the technology of personnel information systems is very flexible, several organisational structures were proposed. However, proposals which entailed dissolution of existing organisational structures and the setting-up of new ones were considered "not feasible" by the upper management. According to the authors, proposals for changes in organisational structure are often opposed because they threaten to affect the established power structure. Moreover, as noted in the Norwegian report, the piecemeal or step-by-step introduction of new technology tends to preserve the existing organisational structure with its departmentalisation and hierarchy.

It is quite understandable that organisations try to maintain a stable situation during the implementation of technological change. In fact, an important lesson from socio-technical research is that technology should build on existing structures, communication patterns and information flow as much as possible. However, this does not mean that organisations ought not to change and that adaptation should be a one-way process. In fact, as described in the Swiss case studies, problems arise when "organisational principles required during the stage of centralised data processing continue to be followed, even though the necessity for them no longer exists". The less-than-optimal results reported underscore the fact that the potential of new technology can only be realised "when existing organisational structures are not seen as unchangeable limits". Otherwise, large and inflexible computer-based systems are likely to reinforce and exacerbate the problems of rigidity in bureaucratic organisational structures, of which they become a central core controlling the network of information.

Implications for jobs

As the relationships between technology and organisation have become more pervasive, complex and subtle, jobs inevitably have changed. Earlier computer systems used large mainframe computers, performed limited distinct functions, relied on batch-processing procedures and were tended by specialised full-time operators. Today, technology is increasingly communication-based; it uses networks and is more comprehensive in terms of the functions carried out within a given system. Large numbers of managers, professionals, administrative and clerical personnel use computers as part of their work. Thus, the new systems have affected more and more jobs. Some jobs have disappeared, some jobs have been created, some jobs have been merged, and some jobs have become routine while others have been enriched.

There have been considerable variations in the type and degree of effects on jobs depending on the category of workers concerned, the characteristics of the organisation, the type of technology introduced and the process of introduction. The most important effects described in the reports relate to work content and the quality of working life: autonomy, responsibility and control; skill requirements and career opportunities; relationships with co-workers and clients; and work pressure.

Several of the national reports were rather pessimistic about the overall effects on jobs in spite of improvements in certain job characteristics or dimensions. Some authors believe that new technology tends to accentuate Taylorist-style restructuring, characterised by deskilling, decreased control over one's job, disrupted or ambiguous career structures and work stress. Women workers are particularly affected.

10

Autonomy and responsibility on the job

One of the most noticeable effects of many computer systems is that the discretion and autonomy exercised by individuals within the organisation may be reduced. Significant areas of decision-making which were previously the responsibility of the individual can be taken over by the computer, or centralised in specialised departments or head offices. For example, according to the reports, marketing and sales managers in the Federal Republic of Germany, Japan and the United Kingdom had lost their responsibility for pricing, negotiating with suppliers and determining sales or special promotions. Moreover, the feelings of loss of autonomy and responsibility of British departmental managers were compounded by a "widespread inability to use the comprehensive analyses produced by head offices to guide them". Examples are also given of clerks, tellers and administrative staff in banks, insurance companies and offices in general whose autonomy and responsibilities were curtailed when areas in which they had previously been able to make decisions were programmed into the computer, leaving them simply to key in data and to transmit machine-produced calculations and analyses. The British report also describes how some banks are currently developing branch information systems based on customer data captured when accounts are opened and updated. There is a real possibility that credit-scoring techniques based on customer files will replace the personal judgement of managers and loan officers over the approval of loans. The Japanese report describes how traditional programming work in the software business has been replaced by so-called "structured programming". One of the goals of structured programming was "to eliminate personal differences in programming". The previous practice wherein programmers structured programmes differently, according to their preferences, with the same end result, was considered inefficient. Structured programming allows all programmes to be built from a small number of specified basic units.

However, properly designed computerised systems have maintained, if not increased, the autonomy and responsibility of some jobs, while also providing the advantages of increased access to information. For example, the introduction of POS terminals in some Japanese department stores made it easier for sales assistants to respond immediately to customer enquiries. Moreover, operating the terminal was just a minor part of the jobs of sales assistants and did not change the practice of allowing groups of assistants under section supervisors to decide on their respective tasks among themselves. The report from the Federal Republic of Germany also describes how rationalisation and new technology improved the work content of "qualified specialists" by increasing the number of independent decisions (e.g. concerning loans and credit), by widening the spectrum or scope of tasks or by enabling them to concentrate on complicated cases. This was made possible because of the nearly total computerisation of simple processes such as calculation, registration and checking and because of the ease of access to up-to-date information. In the United Kingdom, on-line terminals were preferred to batch processing because such terminals enabled bank staff "to control the organisation of their work" in order to decide, for example, when to deal with intermittent entries like amendments and requests.

The reactions of different workers to the degree of autonomy and responsibility remaining in their jobs after technological and organisational changes are also discussed in some of the country reports. For example, an opinion poll carried out by the Japanese Federation of Electrical Machine Workers' Unions in 1982 showed that workers satisfied with their work tended to emphasise the "opportunities given them to carry out their ideas". In the Swiss report, dialogue systems which were flexible and allowed the user to make choices concerning procedures were given a more positive rating by users. In the United Kingdom, part-time cashiers report that they now have less freedom to choose their own method of working and less knowledge of how well they have done their work. On the other hand, nurses in intensive care units, who derived an unusual amount of authority from their observation and care of the patient and their familiarity with complex cases, did not consider that the introduction of computerised patient monitoring systems undermined their position and responsibility.

Skill requirements and training

Much of the debate about the impact of new technology focusses on its implications for the skill requirements of jobs. Specifically, there is disagreement as to whether new technology tends to promote the deskilling or upgrading of jobs.[2] One view is that new technology deskills through increased fragmentation, specialisation and formalisation of work. Another viewpoint maintains that technology fosters variety, responsibility and skill acquisition.

However, assessment of the impact of new technology on skills is difficult. First, the definition of the concept of "skill" is problematic. For example, criteria for skill evaluation could differ between general vs. specific skills, technical vs. social, or individual vs. collective. Second, a differentiation must be made between tasks, jobs and individuals. It is possible for a particular task to be deskilled, without deskilling the overall job. New or better tasks can be added to the job, or different, but not necessarily higher-level, skills may be required with the use of new technology.

Several examples of deskilling, especially at the lower levels of the hierarchy, are described in the country reports. Using computers for checking, correspondence and calculation in credit institutions and insurance companies in the Federal Republic of Germany resulted not only in fewer employees doing this "subsidiary work" but also in the relatively few remaining workers being mainly concerned with data input activities and the transmission of machine-produced analyses and special "non-computerisable" cases. The Japanese study on banking noted that tellers previous tasks of reconciling the cash balance with the day's record, compiling statistical tables and processing related transactions were now unnecessary. Some traditional clerical tasks have also been absorbed into the system, and tellers and clerks, who are mostly women, now operate terminals during a substantial portion of their working day. In the United Kingdom, the introduction of automated laboratory machines has replaced the scientific, craft-based skills of traditional chemistry techniques and graphreading with the technical skill of scanning large batches of numbers and error messages. Details of particular technical tasks will vary according to whether the auto-analyser is based on the continuous flow principle or that of centrifugal force, but at the analysis stage the technician will basically be engaged in feeding the machine and monitoring the analysis process. At present, the use of automated laboratory analysis appears to have "removed much of the skill and knowledge contained in the three years of education required for the technician (Medical Laboratory Scientific Officer) qualification. Some technicians feared that they would become machine operators". In Japan, the use of structured programming in software development resulted in programmers needing a "narrower range of knowledge than before" to perform their job.

The increasing need for highly educated and skilled staff for certain jobs is cited in many of the country reports. In Finland, for example, the main shortage in the service sector is of highly educated staff in the fields of computer systems design and software development and marketing. In the Federal Republic of Germany, the qualification structure has shifted since the mid-1970s in favour of employees with advanced training in data processing, business consultancy and organisational behaviour. This is particularly true in banking where there is a move towards integrated customer advisory services and the expansion and diversification of credit and investment facilities. In Hungary, where terminals are used most extensively for foreign exchange transactions, dealers who carry out such transactions are required to have a university-level degree in economics as well as fluency in one of the major international languages.

However, it is important to note that specified skill requirements may not be relevant in the performance of a job. For example, as noted in the Hungarian report, the "commercial skilled worker" qualification required for the job of shop assistant is unrelated to the use of POS terminals, the major task of the job. In some cases, there may be differences in the evaluation of various personnel groups concerning the skill requirements of office jobs. For example, in the Norwegian report, personnel in management positions emphasised "traditional office competence", while office workers stressed specific technical qualifications and a "wider conceptual mastery of computer systems". Moreover, it seemed that people in higher organisational positions systematically gave lower estimates of qualification requirements than did the office workers themselves.

There also have been instances of general skill upgrading. Some computer systems have removed much of the drudgery of routine work, and their users greatly appreciate the resulting freedom and opportunity to do more interesting and challenging work. In Norway, for example, the introduction of new technology resulted in each worker being responsible for all customers in a particular geographical area; this required workers to increase their skills and knowledge of the overall process.

Some of the country reports describe the simultaneous upgrading of some jobs and the deskilling of others. This polarisation of skills was attributed to the way work was organised. According to the Norwegian authors, the division of labour had been determined when the software was developed. The companies which they investigated did not purchase pre-packaged programmes but designed their own programmes to suit their particular requirements. Planners and system designers had specified who could have access to particular information and who would use specific systems. Similarly, the reorganisation which led to better jobs and higher skills occurred when it became an explicit goal or policy of the company. This perspective is reiterated by the British authors in their case studies which showed that "job content does not change along single trajectories of upskilling and deskilling".

A recurrent concern in the country reports was that polarisation will reinforce and extend the division of labour wherein women's jobs – which are usually at the lower levels of the hierarchy – are deskilled, and men's jobs – which are usually supervisory, managerial or professional – are upgraded. It is clear that while some women may be able to take advantage of the opportunities presented by new technology to move into higher-level jobs, as noted in the case studies of British department stores, it is likely that the majority will remain in the lower levels of the polarised hierarchy and may even face further deskilling with advances in technology.

Due to changes in organisational structure, jobs, and skill requirements, training has often been cited as an important priority. The main point made in the various country reports, however, is that training is often superficial and insufficient. For example, in Norway, the most common form of training is limited to how to use the visual display terminal, word processing system or POS terminal. Such training is usually restricted to employees who will use the system daily in their work. Concerning the duration of training, in Japan, a supermarket manager indicated that the initial training period for newly hired cashiers had been shortened from three days to one day. Most vendors are also constantly trying to shorten the duration of the training period, so that in some cases it lasts only 30 minutes.

Moreover, as noted in the Norwegian study, the training provided under the purchase agreement for single-user units covered only one person who was subsequently expected to train co-workers. Problems arose because the short course given by the vendor often did not qualify the person to train others adequately. Finding the time to train others was another problem.

Self-training in the form of self-teaching programme packages is increasingly becoming a common mode of training. But there are problems with teaching oneself. Many workers are not allowed training time on the job and in the cases where it is allowed they often have problems "getting the necessary peace and quiet", as noted in the Norwegian study. In addition, the manuals and reference material used to familiarise workers with the overall computer system were often found to be difficult to understand and, therefore, were used rarely.

One Norwegian company, however, set a positive example. An internal course, consisting of a general introduction to computers linked to an introduction to the specific computer system used in the company, was designed for all employees. In addition, the course covered health, ergonomics and the work environment, as well as the legal and regulative framework. The company's computer experts designed and gave the course, asking external lecturers to contribute to it, when necessary. The course was comprehensive and at the same time specific to the activities of the company. It was not reserved or limited to specific groups but was open to all employees. An effort was made to link the course to an individual's work and employees were encouraged to ask questions and exchange experiences.

Career opportunities

Changes in job content and organisational structures influence career mobility within organisations as well as in the external labour market. In many countries, career prospects for staff, especially those at the lower levels, have been adversely affected by the introduction of new technology. Computerised systems have sometimes led to the truncation of internal job ladders, because tasks and jobs that might have provided intermediate rungs have been automated and because the simplification and routinisation of some tasks has meant that workers have to learn only a small part of the overall work. This makes the worker less valuable to the employer or organisation, since she or he can easily be replaced by others who require minimum training, or have learned the same simple procedures in other firms. For example, according to the British report, the polarisation of jobs has generated the view in the banking sector that "what is now ... required for clerical staff is a basic level of training, sufficient for their limited role and which does not raise false expectations that they will progress to holding positions of responsibility as 'bankers'". It is, therefore, not surprising that many workers, especially clerical and non-specialist administrative staff, found that their expectations of improving their qualifications and jobs had partly been "wishful thinking", as noted in the Finnish study. In several instances, workers have gone to other firms or have started their own businesses rather than wait for a promotion.

However, the introduction of new technology also has opened new career paths for some categories of workers. The Japanese report cited a study by the National Federation of Electrical Machine Workers' Unions of two large data-processing companies which indicated that software developments had made the demarcations between system engineers and programmers, as well as between programmers and computer operators less rigid and more permeable. Workers can be promoted according to both seniority and ability. However, it was uncertain whether promoting operators to programmers was common practice in smaller data-processing companies and in other industries. Case studies of supermarkets in the United Kingdom showed that the introduction of EPOS (electronic point-of-sale) terminals led to changes in the career opportunities of shop-floor workers, who could become either chief cashier for the whole store or departmental manager, a position normally occupied by a male.

Work pressure

Computerisation of the work process has been associated with increased tension and work pressure. Increased volume of work, time pressure, demand for accuracy, computer breakdowns, performance assessments and intensity of concentration are contributory factors. Tension and work pressure often result in stress and physiological problems.

The computer's capacity to process more information rapidly and the simplification of tasks often lead to increased workload. According to the Finnish study, the pressure of work had increased because the quantity of information to be processed had multiplied: "Much more than before should be accomplished ... at a much faster rate". The Swiss study showed that word-processing operators spent a greater amount of their working time typing than their colleagues using conventional typewriters. The reason for this difference could be attributed to the fact that word-processing operators were often assigned more typing work and that newly introduced word-processing systems acted as "magnets", attracting more typing work. In addition, authors tended to take less care in producing draft texts and increased their demands for revision and correction.

The Japanese report also provides examples of a greater volume of work. Bank tellers behind "high" counters process 200 to 250 transactions from 9:00 a.m. to 3:00 p.m., except during the lunch interval. This means an average work cycle of 90 seconds. The demand by head offices for more data, or more frequent submission of reports from branch offices as part of the process of centralisation of decision-making, has led to an increased volume of work for branch office staff.

In the Swiss study, employees in one company considered the instant accessibility of up-to-date information to be useful but saw this advantage as being offset by "unpleasant extra work", including an increase in the number of administrative procedures required to process information. When questioned about changes in their work since the introduction of dialogue systems, a majority stated that the activity itself had become less difficult but that the work pace, pressures to perform, demands for accuracy and concentration and job stress had increased.

One of the advertised benefits of new technology is that it minimises routine tasks and provides opportunities for more interesting work. Often, this has not been the case. For example, in the Swiss study, the original expectations of employees that work would be less routine were generally not fulfilled due to the workload. Similarly, the prediction that automated laboratory machines would release technicians for more interesting research work was not fulfilled. Despite a reduction in the technician's clerical functions, "the introduction of such machines has been accompanied by a vast increase in workload".

Certain personnel policies and office practices may also lead to an increased workload. For example, employee ratings are widely used in Japanese firms as a means of personnel management. There is "always the possibility that records of terminal operations are used to appraise performance of operators". In fact, one manager stated that he referred to the records of individual operators which indicated the number of cases handled as well as the errors corrected. As noted in the study from the Federal Republic of Germany, the "genuinely epoch-making change in control lies in the fact that by means of the new EDP technology, not only the results of the work but above all its course can be monitored almost totally in its individual stages".

Certain expectations about the capacities of the new technology can exacerbate workload problems. For example, the Finnish report noted that supervisors or managers often had an "unrealistic picture of the limits of a system which they themselves did not directly use". They expected more work to be done more quickly with the new technology. The report from the Federal Republic of Germany describes how, with the computerisation of simple sequences which supposedly facilitates concentration on more complicated cases, employees were expected to make decisions more rapidly.

The effects of work pressure are particularly obvious with VDU workers. A 1983 survey by the Japanese Ministry of Labour showed that 60 per cent of VDU workers complained of eyestrain and 40 per cent complained of stiff shoulders. A similar survey in 1983 by the Japan Federation of Commercial Workers' Unions (JUC) revealed that "poor scheduling of work" and "mental stress" were among the major causes of dissatisfaction among EDP staff. In the Swiss study it was found that persons using a word processor for three or more hours daily reported eye problems, nervousness and pain in the fingers and arms more frequently than those who had spent less time working on the VDU.

Communication among co-workers and with clients

The workplace, especially the office, is a social environment. As technology changes, social relationships at work may also change. Communication and social interaction at work is important to productivity and commitment to organisational goals. Supportive relationships can also buffer the negative effects of stress at work.

18

Organisation of work and the use of technology can either facilitate opportunities for communication and supportive interaction or close off channels. For example, excessive fragmentation and specialisation of jobs may lead to impersonal and apathetic relationships. There is a tendency for workers to spend more and more time interacting with the computer because of the workload and work pressure or because there is no need or opportunity to interact with others. According to the Norwegian report, "organising work in a way that supports co-operation and informal contact between employees at the lower levels is the exception". The report explains that working with the VDU demands concentration. The office worker often uses the VDU, paper and the telephone simultaneously which means that the brain, the eyes, hands and ears are busy. In such cases, one cannot communicate with colleagues. In common situations, such as in word-processing pools, interdependence among co-workers is often greatly reduced or eliminated, and this makes social interaction unnecessary and even difficult.

In some cases, workers develop group strategies to cope with changes in their jobs and relationships. The Finnish report describes how two groups of office workers developed different strategies to cope with organisational and technological changes. The registry office workers formed a very integrated work group and when the technology was introduced they developed a common strategy of withdrawal from the rest of the organisation. While they resented the lack of participation in introducing the changes, their complaints remained within their work group. They maintained their integrated work community and took care of the needs of their clients but isolated themselves from the rest of the organisation. The other group, the secretaries, developed a different strategy. They had not worked as a group and each one had her own room and her own quota of cases. Since there were not enough terminals for each one, they had to queue and take turns in using the system. This created opportunities to express their frustrations about the content and organisation of work and eventually led to a common discussion group. Their strategy was in many ways opposite to that of the registry office workers. In the registry they wanted "to conserve their social community" while the secretaries set a goal of change.

The new computerised systems have also resulted in a new way of communicating with clients or customers. In the Federal Republic of Germany, in order "to operate successfully and to be promoted within the new structure", a different professional behaviour is necessary. It is characterised by quick decision-making and by "a more aggressive communication style with customers and/or suppliers". In the past, an employee's actions were supposed to be reserved and cautious, whereas now there is an "increased emphasis on aggressiveness and willingness to take risks". The Norwegian report also describes how office employees tend to concentrate more on following the prescribed dialogue with the computer rather than on the open dialogue with the client. For example, instead of listening, the employee will interrupt to ask for a name or a number to enter into the computer, sometimes even before the client has even had a chance to say what he or she wants. Some systems may have a dialogue on the VDU where the operator must maintain a certain speed. If the operator does not fill in the next space within a specific time, the display disappears. Consequently, the operator directs the client and controls the way the information is given.

Some of the country reports emphasise that office work is a daily, problem-solving activity where practical knowledge evolves through communication and interaction among co-workers. Office workers are constantly describing and explaining situations to each other. They often tell each other the background of certain activities or the connections between them. In so doing they develop a common understanding of their work and its objectives and thus provide the common framework necessary for procedures and routines to function. Thus the "informal" aspects of office work contribute to the pattern of information processing in addition to facilitating co-operation and goodwill among co-workers.

Technological and organisational choice

One of the main themes of the country reports is that organisations have strategic choices to make in their use of technology. While the technology is increasingly powerful, it is also flexible and capable of being shaped into a great variety of forms with different effects. The range and variation of applications provide dramatic evidence against the "technological imperative". The effects of the technology reflect the way that it has been used rather than any properties inherent in the technology.

Some of the country reports describe the possibility of choice and the implications of these choices for the content of jobs. The Swiss report provides several examples. One case describes the great diversity of organisational structures within the secretariats of the 15 agencies of the federal administration of Switzerland. Specifically, the authors found two extremes in secretariat organisation with the introduction of word processors. In Agency 1, there was strict separation of typing and administration. Typing was done centrally in two word-processing secretariats and administrative tasks were performed in several administrative secretariats. Only secretaries in the word-processing secretariats used word-processors. In Agency 2, eight small secretarial units of two to three employees each were established. The secretariats performed all duties falling under their subdivisions of the agency. The word-processors were at the disposal of all the secretariat employees. Not surprisingly, the secretariat employees rated their possibility for participating in decision-making concerning work as "very little" in Agency 1 to "very great" in Agency 2. The previously-mentioned examples of designing work organisation in a multinational enterprise based in Switzerland and in the secretariats of a federal agency also illustrate the options available.

The British investigation of a regional bank and a clearing bank serves "to qualify any simple view of the so-called 'impact' of new technologies". The introduction of the new technology equipment at the branches was determined centrally together with the operating systems and associated tasks. Even so, the allocation of tasks to jobs (i.e. to particular employee positions) could vary between branches according to the discretion of local management. The potential to modify the organisation of work and the content of specific jobs around a given set of systems and technologies certainly existed. "The same hardware such as counter terminals can be configured and programmed so as to perform different functions, and the content of staff roles can be defined with corresponding flexibility of choice." The study also showed that the general criteria used, which differed in the two banks, were not technologically determined but reflected each management's view of providing service. The clearing bank was moving towards providing a wide range of services to meet the needs of a segmented market, while the regional bank operated in what it regarded as an unsegmented market and offered a fairly standard package of services.

Since the effects on workers depend on decisions concerning design and use of the technology's powerful capacities, the critical question is: Who are the decision-makers? In other words, whose values and interests underlie the choices made?

The Hungarian report notes that top-level managers have a key role in the introduction of new technologies because innovation is an issue of strategic importance to the organisation. In addition, "outside influence, particularly from the upper levels of the ministry, are brought to bear on those at the top level in the organisation". The decision-making process usually consists of approval of the initial concept by top management followed by the submission of a detailed plan.

In Finland, decisions concerning technological changes are often made by managers, although consultants are hired if special expertise is needed. As a rule, office workers are not included in the decision-making process. Where planning is delegated to a special project group, which is quite common in large organisations, office workers are mostly "represented" by their department superiors. According to the author, the implications of decisions and choices for work organisation and the social relationships at work are often neglected because they are not considered as potential problems or because the existing power structure tends to oppose any organisational changes. The employee's right to participate in the planning and control of change remains a politically controversial issue in Finland. The Norwegian report describes a similar situation where managers who do not normally use computer systems have been selected by computer experts "to represent users in project groups".

Relationships between users and technical experts can often be a source of tension. They often have different values and criteria for evaluating success and different perceptions of each other's roles. System engineers may regard users as amateurs, while users may think that they will not receive good tools or systems from people who do not know the business. Such attitudes obviously make co-operation in the design and implementation process difficult.

The reasons why not all the technically available options are considered can be attributed to those who commission the project, according to the Swiss report. This becomes clear at the early stage of planning when improvements in work organisation are rarely recognised as possible goals of the project. In addition, the organisation of the project (e.g. allocation of responsibilities, procedural arrangements) is often unilaterally determined by EDP concerns. Another reason is that departments engage their own EDP specialists to ensure that the new system will fit the existing organisational structure.

Several of the reports suggested that a socio-technical systems analysis from the first stages of project design would permit optimisation of both the technical and the social systems of the organisation. The two systems are so interlinked that changes in one system have consequences and effects in the other. Socio-technical systems design is intended to balance these consequences.

Projects which address only the technical or the social aspects of the organisation, as shown in several of the examples described in the reports, led to increased workload and work pressure, job dissatisfaction and more frequent co-ordination and communication problems. Certain points should be kept in mind in using socio-technical systems analysis in the service sector, particularly in offices: the work flow and structure tend to be less well-defined than in industry; much of the new technology is flexible and locally programmable; and the workforce consists primarily of women but is managed mostly by men.

Implicit in the socio-technical perspective is the idea that there is no foolproof recipe for success. What is needed is a strategy describing the process rather than the outcomes and setting general goals or a range of purposes while leaving the methods to achieve these flexible and adaptable. This strategy should not be improvised but should be based on sound organisational and social as well as technical principles. It should feature explicit values with regard to people and work, clear objectives, realistic and flexible methods and sensible timetables.

New technology is commonly viewed as a mixture of great potential benefits and great potential hazards. In many cases, there is a tendency to oversell the benefits and to evade the problems. The critical issue is choice, or more specifically, conscious selection from available choices. Who makes these choices, and what criteria they use, will determine much of the quality of working life for workers in commerce, offices and health services.

Notes

1   T. Bikson and J.D. Eveland: *New office technology: Planning for people*. Work in America Institute Studies in Productivity (New York, Pergamon Press, 1986).

2   O. Bertrand and T. Noyelle: *The evolution of new technology, work and skills in the service sector* (Paris, OECD, 1986).

2 Step by step: new systems in an old structure

M. LIE AND B. RASMUSSEN

Introduction

This report is based on a research project on the effects of the introduction of computer-based work systems in Norwegian offices.[1] The project was financed by the Ministry of Local Government and Labour and was carried out from 1980 to 1983 at the Institute of Social Research in Industry (IFIM) in Trondheim.

The project is part of a larger, long-term research programme at IFIM on technological change in working life. The overall aim of the programme is to influence the development and introduction of technology by co-operating with the Norwegian Institute of Technology as well as with trade unions. This study of office automation was carried out as part of a research sub-programme on technology, women and work.

Towards the end of the 1970s, computer technologists and information systems experts were forecasting revolutionary changes in office work and employment. Since office workers are predominantly women, the project focused on how women office workers experienced the introduction of new computer technology in offices and to what extent they could influence systems development and the use of computers in their work.

The project started with two exploratory studies. The methodology consisted of participant observation, open-ended interviews of management and office workers, group interviews (where preliminary results were discussed) and in-depth studies of selected office situations. Approximately 20 small- and medium-sized companies, representing different kinds of office organisation, were visited during the first pilot study. In each case at least one representative from management and one from the local trade union were interviewed. This provided an overview of the kinds of office technology that have been installed for different kinds of office work, how data systems were introduced, and what plans companies have developed for the future. Additional information was obtained from three companies in the office computer equipment sector, to provide some kind of future perspective.

The second pilot study consisted of interviews with sales representatives from ten companies selling word-processing systems in Norway. The aim was to get a general overview of both the sale and uses of word-processing equipment in Norway and the kind of advice given to client companies.

After the pilot studies were completed, five of the companies were selected for an in-depth study of lower-level office workers. The companies chosen were representative of different types of business and had experienced some degree of participation by the employees.

A trade union course on new technology in the office was also organised.[2] The course lasted one year, with three meetings of one to two days. The aim of the course was to encourage union representatives to formulate strategies regarding new technology and to prepare them for participation in the planning process.

General background

Since the business community is dominated by small enterprises, workplaces are extensively decentralised in Norway. Office functions tend to be specialised but not centralised, and large office units, such as typing pools, are the exception.

Working life in Norway is regulated by a network of laws and agreements. Norway has a highly centralised, co-operative system of industrial relations. The most important regulations are the Work Environment Act (1977), the Industrial Democratization Act (1973) and the Basic Agreement negotiated between representatives of the National Confederation of Unions (LO) and the Norwegian Employers Federation (NAF). Trade union membership is high in all sectors of labour. Most labour unions belong to the National Confederation of Unions (LO), which occupies a central position in the political system through its close connection to the Labour Party (Norway's largest political party). The LO has been influential in the implementation of the network of laws and regulations governing employment and redundancy conditions, the work environment and democratisation of working life.[3] The laws and agreements are comprehensive and regulate most aspects of working life, such as health and safety, psychosocial factors and company development.

Agreements similar to the one between the LO and the NAF are also found in the public sector. The Union of Clerical Workers is one of the weaker unions but is nevertheless governed by all joint agreements between the LO and the NAF.

Negotiations on wages and working conditions are either centralised with the authorities participating in drawing up a joint framework agreement, or carried out by the different national unions individually. Within the general national framework or branch agreement, the union can negotiate for an extension of the national agreement at plant level.

Although the unions are highly centralised, there are independent organisations at plant level. They have the right to negotiate on all issues specified in the Basic Agreement. Apart from negotiating, the unions also appoint representatives to co-operative committees specified in the Work Environment Act.

The introduction of new technology is regulated by law as well as by the Basic Agreement. The Work Environment Act (1977) states the following in section 12.3:

> The employees and their elected union representatives shall be kept informed about the system employed for planning and effecting the work, and about planned changes in such systems. They shall be given the training necessary to enable them to learn these systems, and they shall take part in planning them.

The first labour-management agreement concerning computerisation was made in 1975 between the LO and the NAF. This has now been incorporated into the Basic Agreement between the two parties. The most important provisions are the right of employees to be given information and to influence the computerisation process and to elect a shop steward concerned with computers, who is entitled to appropriate training. Some companies have also drawn up supplementary local agreements which specify these rights in more detail.

Research has supported the development of these laws and regulations. Since the 1960s there has been more or less continuous research in areas such as democratisation, worker participation and co-operation in working life and technological change.[4] This research has formed the basis of the new Work Environment Act which obliges companies to establish satisfactory working conditions. A second strong tradition is co-operation with the trade union movement.

The first local agreement concerning computerisation was drawn up in 1974 and was the result of a research project on the consequences of the introduction of new technology, carried out in co-operation with a local branch of the trade union.[5] Research on the consequences of the introduction of new technology has been conducted in a number of projects covering a variety of sectors of the economy.[6] In addition, it has also been concerned with the influence of trade unions.[7]

Laws and agreements provide channels through which trade unions can, in theory, exert influence. They are represented on company boards and internal committees for the work environment and technology.

Women and work

Changes have been occurring in the office sector where women employees are heavily represented.

Women in Norway are working outside the home at an increasing rate. In 1972, 45 per cent of women in the age group 16 to 74 were engaged in paid work, and in 1984 this figure had increased to 59 per cent (compared with 77 per cent of men in the same age group).

The increase in the number of employed women was accompanied by an increase in part-time work. Only 56 per cent of working women work 30 hours or more per week, compared with 90 per cent of the working men. However, part-time work is not particularly widespread in the office sector, and new recruitment consists almost entirely of full-time positions. Part-time positions are usually created at the request of individual workers who have established themselves in the company. Under current conditions, many feel unsure about their chances of getting a full-time position back and are now often reticent about making such requests. Special part-time arrangements have been offered in data entry, particularly when the number of personnel in these departments is being reduced. This means the women are hired on a part-time basis without any assurance of permanent employment. Apart from this, the introduction of new technology does not seem to have influenced part-time employment.

The practice where women worked for a few years before having children and then returned to work when their children were older is no longer typical. In all the companies studied, both staff and management said that it is rare for a woman to resign following marriage or childbirth. This was attributed to the previously mentioned difficulty of re-entering the labour market.

While employment in industry has been steadily decreasing, employment within the public sector and the office sector has been increasing. In 1980, 25 per cent of the working population in Norway were employed in offices. Interviews with companies revealed that new technology was adopted partly in order to limit this growth in number of employees. Companies are interested in using technology to do more work with the same number of employees. Whereas most workplaces increased the number of employees in the 1960s and 1970s, by the end of the 1970s productivity was continuing to increase but employment had levelled off.

The changes that have occurred between 1970 and 1980, partly as a result of new office technology, have reduced the number of employees in areas where women are highly represented. This is particularly the case with women doing "unspecified", that is clerical, work. Employment has increased among professionals and management where the men dominate. Few women have reached these positions, although there is a positive trend.

Increasing numbers of highly educated people are recruited directly to senior positions. These are mostly male graduates with degrees in economics, administration and computer science.

In relative terms there are more positions that require higher education and fewer positions for clerical workers. Many young females take a single year of commercial and clerical studies at the upper secondary school. However, as women holding clerical or secretarial positions now tend to keep their jobs, it has become more difficult for young people to enter such positions. Consequently, there is fairly high unemployment among young females with commercial education.

The educational level in Norway is rather high. Still, there is a marked difference between males and females in the level of education attained.

Office work and computer systems

Data-processing systems were first introduced in Norwegian offices in the 1960s. These were batch systems where punched cards were sent to a central computer (inside or outside the company) to be processed at regular intervals (e.g. once a month). The punching was usually done in a special department on the basis of forms filled in by clerical workers. The office workers would then get updated datasheets in return once or twice a month.

By the end of the 1970s, more powerful and cheaper data-processing systems with "intelligent" terminals and visual display units (VDUs) and on-line connections to a central computer were available. These new machines and systems replaced the older systems, and the use of microprocessors had made it economically interesting to develop systems for new functions in the office.

When word-processing systems were introduced, there were forecasts of a revolution in the office where data- and word-processing systems would be connected to create a "paperless office". This meant that firms would be highly involved in acquiring integrated systems and looking for connections between data- and word-processing systems. Our investigation, however, did not indicate a trend towards an integrated, "paperless" office. Only a quarter of the companies had started using word-processing equipment and these tended to be used as advanced typewriters.[8]

Interviews with suppliers of word-processing equipment likewise confirmed this finding.[9] They reported a steep increase in sales from 53 machines in 1977 to over 600 in 1980, but this figure was still not high enough to be talked of in terms of a "revolution in the office". Most of the equipment sold or leased was in the form of stand-alone machines.

Interviews with suppliers showed that most word processors were sold to universities, research institutions and public agencies. These organisations were interested in word-processing equipment to produce lengthy documents and reports which require extensive correction. In companies stand-alone machines were used for specific tasks, such as the updating of price lists and lists of addresses. Normal typewriters were used for correspondence.

The use of computer systems for numerical calculations (data processing) was much more extensive, and all the companies except one had on-line systems with VDUs. This coincided with a Norwegian investigation which found that while 10 per cent of office workers used word processors, 45 per cent used data processors.[10] Though we discovered no revolution in the office as far as word-processing systems were concerned, major changes were in progress in the area of data processing. New computer systems were being introduced for an increasing number of work operations. Batch-type systems were being replaced by on-line systems, and VDUs replaced the monthly computer print-outs. At the end of 1980, over half of the companies investigated employed on-line systems, and many more had plans to start to use such systems in 1981.

Most companies used computers for wage calculations and accounting. In addition, private companies had their customer index, order processing and stock control systems linked to their invoicing system.

The reasons for starting to use computer systems varied: information is easily accessible and more up-to-date; customers receive better and quicker service; better statistics and increased access to information provide a basis for improved planning; and double data registration is eliminated. In addition, stock control can be improved with less capital tied up in warehouse stock, since invoices can be forwarded sooner and customer payments received earlier.

What is office work?

To understand the process of computerisation in the office, one must clarify the special nature of office work. The specific duties of clerical workers vary from company to company and from office to office. In general, clerical work consists of receiving, sorting, systematising and checking communications, and answering inquiries.

Clerical workers usually deal with large quantities of forms (e.g. purchase or sales orders, communications from customers, etc.). Work which formerly consisted of filling in forms is increasingly done on VDUs.

Though these tasks are usually considered routine, there is a fairly extensive degree of judgment involved. The information is seldom uniform, yet it must be uniform to be registered on the computer system. To do this correctly and efficiently requires experience. If the work were purely routine, anyone would be able to do it after receiving concise instructions. It is evident that experience is needed because those with the most experience get the most responsible work, for example, entering information which concerns large sums of money. Judgment is also required to interpret incoming information, which may be in the form of a written communication, or a written or oral inquiry.

An important part of the work is providing services connected with the transfer of internal and external information. Office staff must be able to interpret incoming inquiries, combine them with their knowledge of the information which has been stored and obtain the information required. The ability to handle people is also an asset.

We have extrapolated four recurrent elements in the various tasks of clerical workers. This gives an idea of the types of skill they often need to carry out their work:

- knowledge of administrative systems and routines;
- knowledge of the company;
- integrative ability, that is, ability to interpret inquiries and to improvise when routine and standard operating procedures fail to cover all eventualities;
- ability to offer service and to handle people.

These skills are usually acquired by women from their work experience and in the process of socialisation. Prokop[11] has described how women acquire the ability to relate, to understand and to attempt to satisfy

31

the needs of others as they grow up. Their socialisation makes them particularly well suited to service occupations. It is taken for granted that women will have particular characteristics and skills, such as providing service and keeping things orderly. A certain knowledge is assumed, although it is not asked for and is not included in any training programme. The skills are not valued in the same ways as skills that have been formally acquired. As women are expected to have this knowledge, it is not recognised as occupational knowledge. The result is that the part of their work which requires these skills becomes invisible and the work is termed "unskilled".

This "invisible" element in office work is not only intrinsically important, but is also essential if the office is to function. Wynn[12] stressed the importance of the ability to solve problems in office work. Employees acquire their knowledge of how to solve problems through conversation with each other during the course of their daily work. These conversations result in a common basis for interpretation that is necessary not just for procedures but also to get routines to function.

Routine work, learned through the training process, is only one of the four elements in office work that is visible and acknowledged. Knowledge about the company, the line of business, customers and other external connections, on the other hand, are acquired gradually through work experience when dealing with customers and other external contacts. Individual customers do not ask standard questions; each presents particular problems in his or her own way. Thus, employees are obliged to become involved with complex procedures and to exercise discretion.

New employees are usually given only basic knowledge of the routines during a short training period. Lengthy experience, therefore, is required before one can work independently without making mistakes. Routine instructions can never cover each and every situation and must be adapted to specific cases.

These four different elements are thus related, each one constituting a prerequisite for the next. When computerisation occurs, the *visible* part of the work – that is, the *manual routines* – are computerised. The result is that the manual office routines require less skill, and service work, which is less tangible, requires relatively more skill.

Consequently, the area of work which expands most is the direct provision of service to customers. Before, storage and recovery of information took the most time; today, more time is available to provide information.

Conflicting requirements: Flexibility and co-ordination

The introduction of computers is only part of the general development in the office sector, being one of many ways of working more effectively with large quantities of information. The current transition to modern computer systems is a social process which builds largely on the existing structure of offices. Computer sytems are introduced piecemeal for a single isolated function, in department after department. This step-by-step computerisation process preserves the existing organisational structure with its departmentalisation and hierarchical organisation. The objective of each computer system is to make existing tasks or functions more effective.

Word-processing equipment is purchased and used independently from data-processing systems. Furthermore, for systems which are constructed in the form of interchange between departments, i.e. for linked operational tasks, each sub-system tends to be designed individually. Thus, design is on a departmental basis and systems are dedicated to limited functions within each individual department.

Consequently, a company is almost never "fully" computerised. Considerable variation was found between departments of the companies studied. Some office routines were computerised, others were not. In some cases the system worked satisfactorily, in others it did not. One of the main reasons behind these differences is that organisations are divided up into a number of different departments in order to carry out a range of dissimilar tasks. It cannot be expected that a system which functions in one procedural context, and is designed to meet the specific requirements of one department, will be equally suitable in other departments.

As well as the introduction of flexible departmental computer systems, there is a need for co-ordination. Communication between departments can be facilitated by more extensive and co-ordinated use of computers. The accounting system has a key role to play in this context. Most companies started using computers in accounting systems, and then all other departments in the company were obliged to produce data to be processed in the accounting system. Efficiency in the office is greatly increased by linking the registration of orders and accounting. Thus, once the order is registered by the sales representative or by the orders department, the invoice is written out automatically and the sum registered in the accounting system and, if applicable, also in the customer's account.

The companies were therefore faced with two conflicting requirements: flexible adjustment to the dissimilar demands of the different departments and the demands of co-ordination.

The advantages of the co-ordinated system have been stressed by computer experts and in predictions concerning the future of offices. When companies proceed step-by-step and opt for individual systems, this is held to be indicative of their conservatism and poor planning.

This piecemeal planning and mode of introduction is related to something characteristic of office work: it is difficult to standardise. Specific designs for different tasks in the company are required, and this results in a fragmented organisational structure. The introduction of the new computer system builds upon this tradition.

The purchase price, the problems raised by restructuring, and employee resistance are additional factors that contribute to this cautious step-by-step approach. The most important reason, nevertheless, is that in this way one maintains the complexity that is so characteristic of office work. The development towards smaller machines may lead to a total re-evaluation of the picture that was current at the end of the 1970s, that of a central computer controlling all the functions of the office.

Computerisation: A lengthy, piecemeal process

A number of models have been made of the planning and introduction of computer systems. These models usually build on a division into different phases, as indicated in figure 1.

Figure 1   Stage-by-stage planning and introduction of computer systems

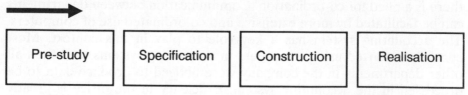

This stage-by-stage approach to project work is the one which is favoured by computer staff. It stresses the importance of planning and of a pre-study. It is considered unwise to start directly with system specification (or to purchase a ready-made system) prior to establishing the need. The division into phases makes it possible to make an assessment after each phase to determine whether to proceed, make alterations, postpone or stop the project.

The way it really works in practice can be illustrated in figure 2.

Figure 2   Stage-by-stage planning in practice

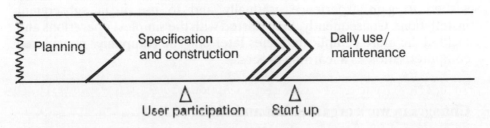

Figure 2 differs from the model of the recommended approach (phase model) in a number of ways. The introduction is a process without separate phases, and there are no definite starting or stopping points in the process.

The reason why the starting point of the project cannot be determined is that planning commences prior to a definite pilot project. It is impossible to state exactly when a company starts to consider plans for the introduction of computers. When someone starts to think along such lines, development starts to take shape and decisions are made. At this stage, the steps taken by management before a definite planning or pilot-project phase has begun are decisive in the long term.

It is also difficult to isolate the end of a computer project. Most literature on computers only treats the phases up to and including the installation. Thus, the project is considered finished when the computer system is made operational. Funds and expertise are allocated by companies for the phases prior to the installation, and the start-up of a system acts as a signal to commence work on a new one. In reality, one is never finished with a system, as there will always be the need for follow-up, adjustments and maintenance. As the life expectancy of computer systems is short (five to ten years), users will have to start with new systems several times in their working careers.

A final point is that it is very difficult to segregate the phases clearly during work on a project. The difference between the distinct phases planned for and the more diffuse process that occurs in reality is usually caused by the fact that there are a number of projects in process in a particular company at any one time, causing interruptions in implementation schedules or delays due to work taking longer than planned.

The companies we studied did not plan one comprehensive computer system to encompass the whole firm. Instead, they planned for each specific function. The companies said that they did this because they wished to gain experience gradually and to use it in subsequent installations. Consequently, they started with the simplest operations and tackled the more complicated ones later on. The companies considered computerisation as a learning process.

Changes in work organisation and skills

Skills

The concept of skills that we use is linked to the content of work. By skills we mean the knowledge and abilities that are necessary to perform a particular job.

Our concept of skill is not linked to education or the job market. The literature on the effect of technological change on skills has mainly centred on whether the level of skills has been raised or lowered. If education were used as a measure, it would seem that the level of skills has been raised because the level of education is rising. It would be just as misleading to use the market as a measure. Since there is a constant supply of people with education in commercial and clerical subjects, companies demand such education when employing workers. This disregards the issue of whether people need this education to be able to perform their duties. A definition of skills based on education and the market may conceal changes in skills which are associated with changes in work duties.

The skills needed in office work are mostly acquired through on-the-job training and experience. Office work partly consists of visible functions, such as filling in forms and filing papers: here there are rules to follow, and experienced colleagues have used their experience to establish procedures. However, a fairly large quantity of "invisible work" is also required to be able to carry out these visible functions.

First, there is a good deal of intellectual effort required since the handling of paperwork necessitates both intellectual effort and assessment. Furthermore, knowledge and skills outside the formally defined routines are necessary to make things run smoothly. Finally, office workers have to communicate a good deal of information orally, and for this there are few rules to follow.

Training on the job consists of the acquisition of new skills as well as the development of social abilities. The formal and visible skills required are mainly learned by doing the job under the supervision of colleagues. The level of skill is therefore dependent on the difficulty of the work and is subject to alteration when changes in the work occur.

Skills and work organisation

Investigation of changes in skills associated with computerisation has revealed two opposing trends. On the one hand, there is a trend towards fragmentation of work and greater specialisation.[13] The separation of routine tasks and extensive formalisation have been necessary in the change to computer processing. If this trend continues as computerisation becomes more widespread, the result will be limited, routine work. On the other hand, it is maintained that, with the introduction of computers, routine work will disappear and be replaced by more comprehensive, interesting work for everyone.[14]

From a historical perspective, both sides may be correct. Fragmentation and specialialisation are a result of the initial transition to computers. It is not axiomatic that the next phase, the transition to on-line systems and the widespread use of visual display units (VDUs) will follow the same path as the first phase of computerisation.

It is the way in which work is organised that determines the content of work and skills. However, the choice of work organisation is not unlimited. Some conditions are determined when the machines and software are being developed. Technology is developed with a particular form of work division already in mind.[15] A simple example of this is the word processor, a special computer for processing of text designed to take over from the typewriter. Because of the traditional division of work, a machine with very limited functions is made for women, while men use a general computer.

A number of principles of work division are found in the software. Each employee has access to only a limited part of the company's computer system. This means that, although not everyone needs to have access to all systems, planners have previously defined who can use which

37

system. This definition excludes employees from acquiring new knowledge and performing new tasks. The development of machines and programmes is also connected to the existing traditions of work organisation. The companies studied did not purchase pre-packaged programmes. They developed their own software to suit their particular requirements. The systems were made with specific users in mind. Development of the systems and development of the work organisation were parallel operations.

Most companies made few alterations to their organisation when introducing new computer systems. The systems were developed in accordance with the form of organisation they already had.

We have described the office organisation as being fragmented into functionally specialised departments, within which the work is split up into simple parts. This fragmentation resulted from the growth of offices and from efforts to work more effectively. It was amplified by the introduction of batch computer systems in the 1960s.

Modern office technology does not in itself lead to a further fragmentation of tasks. Rather, it allows the possibility of assembling fragmented tasks into whole operations, because it facilitates the rationalisation of routine operations and gives access to information on the whole work process. When calculations and invoicing are connected to order processing, for instance, control by superiors is very often made superfluous because control is built into the system.

Our research showed that there was a tendency to combine tasks which were previously fragmented. Small departments were changing from being "conveyor-belt" organisations with strict hierarchies to being a group of employees each doing the same complete set of operations. Responsibility for the whole operation does not necessarily mean that there is a higher demand for skill than before. The computer system may make the different tasks easier and dispose of some of the operations, often the most complicated ones, and by making the work more straightforward, departments can do more of the same type of work.

Sometimes the department still kept senior staff responsible for control, even if the system made this unnecessary. Others reorganised and removed hierarchies, for example by making each worker responsible for all customers in one geographical area. This increased the skills of workers, because they had to acquire knowledge of the overall process in order to give customers good service. Computerisation made the already fragmented tasks simpler, or automatic, and the simpler tasks were connected to whole operations. Requalification occurred where this was followed by a decentralisation of responsibility for the work and contact with the public. This kind of reorganisation was not widespread, because it threatened the jobs of superiors, and thereby their positions, and it threatened the positions and tasks of male employees in a female-dominated group. In addition, firms wanted to keep financial control in a few hands.

Thus, reorganisation leading to better jobs and higher skills did not follow from computerisation. It only happened when it became the explicit will and policy of the firm or department.

Change in work content

We have described the computerisation of offices as having led to only minor changes in the tasks of office workers. The level of skills has changed only marginally for employees of companies where there have been no alterations in the division of work and responsibility. A closer look at the work with new computer systems and the skills required showed that some qualitative changes may be of great importance in the future if they are not recognised and dealt with.[16]

The most visible change is the increasing use of VDUs by office workers. The computerisation of routine operations has meant that less time is spent handling paper and more time is spent providing service to people inside or outside the firms. Although many tasks are taken over by the computer, this part of the job is not computerised. The use of a telephone has been steadily increasing, taking more and more of the office worker's time. With less time spent on routine paper work, relatively more time is available to provide customer service.

In office work, "good service" has progressively come to mean quick service: good service is to receive one's answer or have one's order filled immediately. This definition of good service is not what employees think of as good service. They stress the *quality* of information. They want to be able to give customers the information they want, and perhaps also things they did not ask for, or did not even know were available.

In this kind of work women must use their general skills in communicating. As already mentioned, these skills are developed at work through conversation with colleagues and customers, so that eventually a common language suited to the firm, line of business and duties at work is developed. A Swedish study of computerisation in the social security administration showed the importance of these special "professional languages", and how they may be destroyed by the introduction of computer systems.[17] Mastering the language is an important skill for office staff. They need to understand their work and to be able to explain the information provided by the computer system to customers or clients.

To master this work, office workers need daily training in their "professional language". Many computer systems are made without considering this factor. Therefore, they are not constructed in a way that preserves and develops the user's professional skills. In addition, there are some ways in which the various kinds of computer systems may change the dialogue between the office staff and the people requiring their service.

There is a general contradiction between open-ended, natural language and the formalised language used in data processing. Office staff must act as interpreters between these two languages. They must interpret a disordered message and change it into a pattern that makes it clear enough to be answered. They combine information from the customer with knowledge of their work. During this part of the conversation, employees must be open to the customer's way of giving information about the problem and not make a hasty assumption.

Most of the information that the customer or the client wants may be available on the VDU. This can sometimes present problems. For example, since it is convenient to look up the information for the customer as early as possible, the employee will interrupt to ask for a name or a number to enter in the system before the person has even had a chance to say what he or she wants.

Some systems have a dialogue on the VDU where the operator must maintain a certain speed. If the operator does not fill in the next space within the time given, the display on the VDU disappears, and with it the information already entered. With other systems, the operator has to follow an established order of dialogue. Consequently, the employee will direct the client and control the way the information is given.

Many systems, such as those for processing orders, are built on number codes. Previously, a customer would telephone an order, and an office worker would record it on paper or preprinted forms. Systems built on number codes are supposed to shorten the time by training customers to read numbers instead of the names of the items. Only numbers can be entered in the system and if the customers use the names of items, the office worker has to remember or look up the number to be able to enter the order. If the customer says both number and name, it is more difficult for the office worker to follow the dialogue on the VDU. Consequently, office staff prefer to deal in numbers only.

Employees told us that they have as much contact with the customers as before, chatting with them before or after the order is received. However, the part of the conversation connected with the order is now gone. When the products are not mentioned by name, no natural associations are connected with them. Previously, the customer and the employee would exchange information on the products. The employee would inquire about the quality of orders received, suggest other products, etc. The use of numbers eliminates product-related conversation. Only general small talk remains.

These demands of the system – communicating in number codes or following a certain speed and order – conflict with the principles of human conversation. Office staff are obliged to concentrate more on following the prescribed dialogue with the computer than on open dialogue with the customer or client. This means a new type of communication which is focused on "leading" the customers rather than on listening to them.

The changing learning process

An important aspect of the future of office work is the fear that computerisation will lead to less contact between people because information is exchanged via VDUs instead of on a person-to-person basis. However, this had not happened in the offices studied. There was as much contact between colleagues as before, though there was a change in the content of these contacts. Working with a VDU demands concentration, with several senses in use at the same time. The office worker uses the VDU, paper and often the telephone at the same time. This means that the brain, eyes and hands are busy and, at the same time, the ears register sounds. When using a telephone and VDU at the same time, one *has* to be isolated from colleagues. Sometimes this isolation is visible, when the employees use earphones or are placed in small enclosures. With the phone at their ear and the VDU in front of their eyes, they cannot communicate with colleagues.

Previously, there was more paperwork and less service to customers and other departments. When there was a call for information, employees had to leave the phone to go and look it up. Those who called were used to waiting. In this situation one could seek advice and discuss the matter with colleagues. With the new on-line systems, information is available on the VDU and the customer on the phone expects it immediately. Consequently, it is not possible to ask for advice from colleagues. Contact is postponed until the matter is finished.

Concentration at the VDU has changed the basic pattern of social contact. Whereas office staff previously talked to each other while working, today they talk in between concentrated periods of work on the VDU or the telephone. Isolation, therefore, is not considered to be a problem. People still talk to each other. It is the pattern and content of communication that has changed. Communication is more on general topics and less connected to the work. An opportunity for informal learning is thus lost, since work-related conversation is essential for learning about the work and how to do it better.

Organising work in a way that supports co-operation and informal contact between employees at lower levels is the exception. As VDUs contribute to isolating people while they are completing their tasks, organising work to support co-operation and social contact will be all the more important. Few computer systems have been designed in accordance with the content and context of office work, which requires complicated information processing and human relations skills. This could be overcome if computer systems were designed and implemented differently.

Participation and the computerisation process

Systems development and participation

The Work Environment Act and the Basic Agreement between the LO and the NAF stipulate that there must be employee participation in the process of introducing new computer systems. Computer experts are generally positive towards participation, as it results in the design of more appropriate systems. Although computer experts and trade union representatives agree on user participation in principle, their ideas of what it means and how it should be done vary widely.

Many office systems, whether standard packages or specially ordered, do not function according to specification. Expensive changes have been necessary to make them appropriate for the functions they were designed to perform. System developers are therefore increasingly concerned that those who know the work and the requirements of the new systems, i.e. the end users, should participate in the development process. Nevertheless, there were few examples of office workers actually participating in systems design. We found two different strategies of participation, but neither of them reached the ordinary workers who used the systems daily.

The following forms of participation were used:

- Extensive use of formal channels of representation. The companies in question had established committees with employee representation and had written plans stating the rate at which computerisation would take place as well as long-term plans.

42

- Direct contact between system developers and individual groups of users. The system developers took the initiative and defined the type of participation, the phases and the methods to be used.

The companies we visited had either chosen one of these strategies or participation had taken place on two levels simultaneously in different forums and without co-ordination.

Participation as seen by computer experts

The term employed by computer experts is "user participation". This includes all forms of direct participation by future users of a system – everything from formally established project groups to informal exchanges of information between system designers and users. User participation is not frequently practised in working life.

Where user participation was practised, the computer experts of the company had taken the initiative. They selected managers to represent the users in the project groups. Thus, the employees who participated were generally not the real users, as departmental managers do not normally use computer systems in the same way as the office workers in their departments.

The fact that departmental managers were selected says something about the type of ability computer experts sought. Departmental managers have a general picture of the whole department and know a good deal about what is going on in related departments, while office staff have detailed knowledge of their area of work, and this was seen as too limited to be of much value.

Departmental managers have time allocated for such work, as well as the opportunity to acquire know-how in this area. Office workers, on the other hand, are tied to a fixed objective. They have work which must be taken care of daily, as well as a telephone which has to be answered. The planning of work and the revision of work routines fall within a department manager's sphere.

When office workers were involved at all, it was on an informal basis. Those responsible for the development of the system went to the department and talked to employees. Information was collected about their work routines while the system was being developed, and after the system was operational they were asked how it functioned and whether they had any suggestions for changes.

Another hindrance to real user participation in systems design is the less than ideal scheduling of projects. Computer experts recommended

Figure 3   The systems design and development process

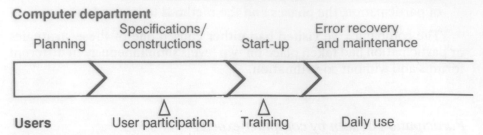

that project specifications should be established prior to the involvement of users, thus providing a clearer definition of the users' tasks.

As figure 3 shows, participation occurs in an extremely limited part of the process. With this form of participation, the purpose is clearly defined: the objective of user participation is to create the most appropriate system possible. The representative is not selected from among colleagues to represent their interests. Issues outside technical system design are not touched on in the computer experts' concept of user participation.

Participation as seen by trade unions

In our investigations we found that trade union participation occurred in other forums and was concerned with issues other than user participation in system design. The shop stewards participated in a computer committee where matters that affected the whole company were discussed. These included planning, the choice of equipment and the consequences for employees as a whole.

As already mentioned, planning commenced on an informal basis long before a formal project was embarked upon. Once a formal plan and a project group are established, a number of assumptions have already been made. Union representatives have little influence on such fundamental decisions as whether or not a company should introduce computers. Furthermore, since the union representative is only able to react to proposals from technical experts, the trade union is always one step behind the planners.[18]

We have described computerisation as a piecemeal process. This piecemeal process affects the work of shop stewards. Department after department receives computer equipment. Systems development, information and training are largely decentralised. Thus, shop stewards have difficulty gaining an overall picture of what is happening. In some companies, project plans and timetables present a coherent picture overall, but in reality they are rather confusing because they are not regularly updated.

The contacts between local computer shop stewards and ordinary union members also posed problems. Shop stewards found it difficult to involve their members in the computerisation process. The members in turn said that they found it hard to form an opinion about something which did not yet exist and which they consequently knew little about. It takes a long time until a project becomes "visible" in a company. Thus, it is only when terminals suddenly appear in a department that the workers can see that something is happening. It is often only then that the reaction and involvement really occur. The result in the companies studied was that people took a "wait and see" attitude. Although they agreed with the principle that the users should be involved beforehand, members felt that they had little to contribute before they had had some experience with computers.

The fragmentary nature of the introduction process and the separate sub-projects for each department sometimes lead to conflicting interests between groups of employees. When a subsystem is introduced in one department, little concern is paid to other departments that will indirectly be affected by it. One department may be satisfied with its computer system because it gives them a better overview, while the same system may create fear and disharmony in another department, because it leaves them with less to do.

Shop stewards considered their role in terms of providing protection for their members, that is, ensuring that the latter did not lose any rights they already had. The result of this strategy was that strong groups among the employees, especially male staff interested in computers, raised their demands and had their interests protected. The shop stewards were less interested in more peripheral groups, e.g. female part-timers or the staff of data-entry departments which are about to be closed down anyway.

Most of the shop stewards elected were male, partially because they were thought to have a better understanding of technology. Frequently, the persons chosen were men who were especially interested in the technical aspects of the computers, and some of them were eventually transferred to the company's computer department. As the computer shop stewards had extensive contact with experts from computer companies, a rapport was established which was essential for both parties. Computer shop stewards learned about computer technology in order to be able to discuss such matters with the company's computer experts. This increased their distance from ordinary employees.

Office workers were interested in knowing about their work situation and work environment. As the shop stewards were not fully conversant with the work and routines of individual departments, it was difficult for the stewards to discuss the systems with those affected. The result was that the shop stewards discussed technical matters and general questions such as computers and employment or the dangers of working with VDUs.

Because of the division in the office between the work of males and females, the male computer shop stewards had little contact with departments which were staffed exclusively by females. Shop stewards frequently characterised women as being uninterested in union matters and unwilling to involve themselves in issues connected with computers until they were suddenly confronted by a VDU on their desks. Trade union representatives considered most of their members to be too short-sighted and uninterested in issues outside their own department. Employees, on the other hand, felt their shop stewards knew too little about the situation in their department to be of any help.

Information received by employees

The computer department was the most important source of information for employees when the new systems were introduced. Office staff received information either in an informal way directly from the computer staff or indirectly through their departmental managers. The degree to which the shop stewards were informed by the company also varied widely.

The information given was mostly restricted to the statement that a new system was going to be introduced, which departments were going to have VDUs and when this would happen. The information given, therefore, merely said that something was going to happen. It provided no answers to the questions the employees were concerned about, such as reorganisation, changes in the work environment, contact between employees and the content of work.

Another channel of information for employees was through their trade union. However, only a minority of ordinary members participated in the computer courses offered by the trade unions. Though the trade unions provided information on the issues employees were concerned about, the computer shop stewards were not familiar with the situation in each individual department, and the information they provided was considered to be too general and abstract.

On the other hand, the information provided on using the new system was more specific and useful. This could be linked to the experience gained from using the system. Employees found that the departmental manager was able to give a more accurate picture of what was happening than the computer shop steward. Traditionally, the departmental managers had the task of keeping employees informed about the situation in the company as a whole and plans that would affect their department. The information from the departmental managers about computers was thus better received as it was concerned with specific issues and was not abstract and general, like the information from the shop stewards.

Training of employees

All the companies using word-processing systems had availed themselves of the limited training offered by vendors. In most cases training lasted two days, in a few cases, three or five days. Our study of vendors revealed that this training period is being shortened constantly.[19] Emphasis is increasingly being placed on self-training in the form of self-instructional programme packages in the word processor. This kind of training is not effective, as operators have problems finding the necessary peace and quiet. Since they are not taken out of the company for training, they have their ordinary work to do at the same time. Another problem is that there is no one to ask for advice. Normally, the training included in the purchase price of single-user units is only for one person, who then is expected to train co-workers. This usually means that a word processor is only operated by the person who has had this training. Moreover, the short course offered by suppliers does not qualify an operator to train others. There is also the problem of finding the time to do so.

The most usual form of training in the use of computer systems was limited to an introduction to the use of the terminal. Individual employees learned the specific functions necessary to complete their tasks. This training usually occurred when the terminal was being installed and lasted from 30 minutes to a few hours. Such training was given to the employees who were to use the system on a daily basis – that is, a single group of employees was trained each time a sub-system was introduced to a department. Information or training was seldom given to all employees. It was restricted to those who were directly affected.

One reason why the training is so brief is that the transition to the new system has to be accomplished without interrupting production. Technical installations were completed outside of working hours. In some cases workers were able to practise on the system for a few evenings or during the weekend before it was made operational. The companies' computer experts generally agreed that prior training had little value, and that training should be linked to the employees' regular work through task-specific training on the terminal. Information on all parts of the system, not just that used on a daily basis, could be found in written form in manuals or reference books. Most employees stated that these were so difficult to understand that they were scarcely used.

In short, training was restricted largely to an introduction to the use of the terminal. Some companies also had pre-packaged courses giving a general introduction to data processing. The problem with this type of training was that there was no connection between the specific user training and the general introduction to computers. The employees had problems assimilating this general knowledge when it was not linked to their own experience with their company's computer system. Some big companies offered a broader introduction to their system, but only those in key positions were sent to such courses.

The computer staff was aware that some employees, particularly the older ones, feared not being able to master the new equipment. Consequently, the transition was simplified as much as possible. Information was restricted to practical information about the type of equipment that was going to be used, while training consisted of learning to use it. This kind of oversimplified information and training makes technology appear harmless. Within a short space of time something that is enormous and unknown is transformed into something that is tangible and simple to understand. As a consequence, this form of information and training fails to create inquisitiveness and to motivate people to learn more. The employees who learned word processing often failed to learn how to use the additional possibilities offered by the system. Most used it as an advanced typewriter with easy correction possibilities and, consequently, they were disappointed by the new machines.

One company did, however, set a positive example by holding an internal course which was designed for all employees. This course consisted of an introduction to all parts of the company's computer system, linking this to a general introduction to computers. In addition, it included issues such as health, the work environment and the legal and regulative framework. The course was planned and held by the company's own computer experts, supplemented by external lecturers. The course gave an overall picture but at the same time it was specific and appropriate to the particular place of work. It was not reserved for specific groups who used the particular parts of the computer system but was open to all employees. Furthermore, the course could be linked to an individual's work experience. Specialists were present so that employees could ask questions and exchange experiences.

Training for participation

The introduction of a computer system creates a need for training as well as an interest in being trained. This could be exploited to give employees a thorough training in the company's total computer system and the possibilities it represents. If this is not done, the ability of employees to participate in improving the systems and to influence the introduction of new systems is very limited.

The daily use of computers helped employees overcome their initial scepticism and fear of computers. Nevertheless, the information and training they had received was insufficient for them to be able to participate in the design of the systems and their working conditions. Management tended to regard computerisation as a learning process in which the experience gained from each sub-project could be used to plan and implement the next project more effectively. Few employees, however, participated in this cumulative learning process, and it was insufficiently focused on issues that concern them most, i.e. training and information.

There was a large gap between the companies' aims of effective transition and change and the training of the employees. Since the computer experts presented the changes linked to computerisation as minor, simple and without any particular consequences, office workers were discouraged from learning and finding out more about computers and the possibilities they provided.

We have presented computerisation as a long-term incremental process. It is not completed when the system is installed. There will be changes and employees will always be presented with the challenges of participation and influence. Today they have the right to participate, but without real influence. The way in which companies and computer experts manage the computerisation process and training programmes will influence the long-term process of participation. Thorough and more extensive training which is *not* reduced to learning one simple routine task is required. This will also give office workers a basis for participation that leads to influence.

Conclusions

New office technology creates possibilities for improving the working environment and developing the skills of office workers, provides more information and simplifies time-consuming routine work. However, most new computer systems are designed with a very limited view of the nature of office work and an uncritical acceptance of the existing organisational structure based on a hierarchical distribution of tasks.

To understand the consequences of office computerisation, the nature of office work has to be understood. Paper flow and office routines are visible to the outsider and are usually easily quantified, but they represent only a part of office work.

There has been a growing concern among office computer experts about the participation of users in developing better systems. More unions are negotiating for the right of workers to participate in implementing computer systems. Clerical workers are not recognised as having the knowledge necessary to participate in decisions about the new systems, but limited worker participation impedes fundamental organisational changes which could improve both effectiveness and job satisfaction. Everyone seems to agree on the need for future users to participate in the computerisation process. There are different ideas, however, as to what participation is, which issues are critical for users and who should participate. Therefore, new office technology tends *not* to improve the working environment or workers' skills and effectiveness.

In designing office systems, computer experts have mainly dealt with the visible parts of office work, i.e. the administrative routines and paper flow. Hence only part – and perhaps not the most significant part – of office work is considered in systems design.

An important and substantial part of the work of office workers is servicing customers and other departments in the firm. The skills needed in such service work are an ability to communicate with customers and to understand their needs, and concrete knowledge of the products, the firm and the industry. The skills and knowledge needed are learned on the job by doing the work and communicating with more experienced colleagues. Unless this learning process is taken into account in developing office computer systems, the systems lead to less effective organisation and a poorer quality of office work.

Unless consciously planned otherwise, office computerisation tends to deskill clerical workers. Less qualified workers will not be able to provide service to customers as well as before and will therefore be less valuable to their firm. The danger is that *computers will make office work more efficient but less effective*.

The tendency to computerise offices on a piecemeal basis is likewise contributing to the deskilling of office workers. The usual process is to introduce single, well-defined functions one at a time. This preserves the organisational structure in offices, including the sex-segregated division of labour. Computer technology creates an opportunity to integrate tasks within and between functions and to upgrade office work, but these opportunities are rarely used. Companies rarely take advantage of the possibilities that new technology creates to widen and enrich the tasks and give clerical workers a greater range of learning possibilities. A redistribution of tasks and planned job development could eventually lead to greater internal mobility and better chances for advancement for female clerical workers.

Developing good systems – systems that increase effectiveness and job satisfaction – is not simply a question of choosing the right technical experts. Participation by the workers who do the work daily is necessary. This requires organisation and training. One must think of participation in new and different ways and organise it accordingly. It can be done, by focusing on clerical workers as skilled workers, and by organising relevant adult education.[20] Clerical workers who are properly mobilised can be "their own best consultant".[21] With changing technology, the computerisation of offices will be an on-going process. It is therefore a good investment to develop clerical workers' ability to participate in continuous self-directed learning as a basis for participating more effectively in the continuous process of change of office computerisation

Notes

1   M. Lie and B. Rasmussen: *Can office work be automated?* [in Norwegian] (Trondheim, IFIM, 1983).

2   H. Finne and B. Rasmussen: *Strategic competence and learning from experience* (Trondheim, IFIM, 1982).

3   See B. Gustavsen and G. Hunnius: *New patterns of work reform: The case of Norway* (Oslo, Universitetsforlaget, 1981)

4   F. Emery and E. Thorsrud: *Democracy at work* (Leiden, Martinus Nyhoff, 1976); M. Elden: "Three generations of work-democracy experiments in Norway", in C.L. Cooper and E. Mumford (eds.): in *The quality of working life in Western and Eastern Europe* (London, Associated Business Press, 1979); Gustavsen and Hunnius, 1981, op.cit.;

5   K. Nygaard and B.T. Bergo: "Trade unions – New users of research", in *Personnel Review* (Epping), Vol. 4, No. 2, Spring 1975, 5-100.

6   M. Elden et al.: *Good technology is not enough* (Trondheim, IFIM, 1982).

7   L. Schneider and C. Ciborra: *Technology bargaining in Norway* (Boston, Harvard Business School, 1983).

8   A. Pape and K. Thoresen: *Word processing – A revolution in the office or new typewriters?* [in Norwegian] (Oslo, Norwegian Computing Center, 1982).

9   L. Schneider: *Words, words, words. How word processing vendors sell their wares in Norway* (Trondheim, IFIM, 1982).

10 MPI (Norwegian Institute of Productivity): *A arbeide pa konter* [To work in an office] (Oslo, NPI, 1980).

11 V. Prokop: *Weibliche Lebenzusammenhang* (Frankfurt A/M, Sulvkamp, 1976).

12 E. Wynn: *Office conversation as an information medium* (Berkeley, University of California, 1979).

13 H. Braverman: *Labor and monopoly capital* (New York, Monthly Review Press, 1974).

14 E. Mumford and D. Henshall: *Participative approach to computer system design: A case study of the introduction of a new computer design* (London, Associated Business Press, 1979); and J. Taylor: *Word processing jobs and organisations* (Geneva, ILO, 1979).

15 M. Lie et al.: *The significance of technology for women's work*, Working Paper (Trondheim, IFIM, 1983).

16 M. Lie and B. Rasmussen: "Office work and skills", in A. Olerup et al.: *Women, work and computerization* (Amsterdam, North Holland Publishing, 1985).

17 B. Göranzon et al.: *Job design and automation in Sweden* (Stockholm, Center for Working Life, 1982).

18 L. Schneider and C. Ciborra: *Technology bargaining in Norway* (Boston, Harvard Business School, 1983).

19 L. Schneider, op. cit.

20 See, for example, Werner Fricke: "Participatory research and the enhancement of workers' innovative qualifications", in *Journal of Occupational Behaviour* (Chichester), Vol. 4, 1983.

21 M. Elden: "Three generations of work-democracy experiments in Norway", in C.L. Cooper and E. Mumford (eds.), op. cit.; and M. Elden: "Client as consultant: Work reform through participative research" in *National Productivity Review* (New York), Vol. 2, No. 2, Spring 1983, 136-147.

3 Computer-aided office work: concepts and research findings

"COMPUTER-AIDED OFFICE WORK" RESEARCH GROUP, WORK AND ORGANISATIONAL PSYCHOLOGY UNIT, SWISS FEDERAL INSTITUTE OF TECHNOLOGY *

Introduction and overview

The work one does affects one's sense of well-being and develops one's personality. Thus, changes occurring within the work environment inevitably have far-reaching consequences for those involved.

Research in organisational and industrial psychology is concerned with establishing the groundwork for the analysis, evaluation and design of humane work and organisational structures. The basic aim is expressed in the following definition of a humane work activity:

An occupation can be designated as humane when it is not damaging to the psycho-physical health of the worker, when it does not – or does only temporarily – impair his psycho-social well-being, when it corresponds to his needs and qualifications, makes possible individual and/or collective influence on the conditions and systems of work, and when it contributes to the development of his personality in the sense of broadening his potentials and increasing his competence.[1]

Up until now, concepts from organisational and industrial psychology have been taken into consideration only to a limited extent in the design of office work. Achieving the optimum in the technical components of the system tends to be seen as the primary goal; psycho-social and organisational aspects are often neglected. This frequently results in job strain for workers, and also leads to increased division of labour which, in turn, leads to lower skill requirements and a general drop in quality. This is so in spite of the fact that electronic data-processing technology exists today which would allow the creation of work systems and organisational structures adapted to human needs and qualifications in a way that was not possible with earlier EDP systems.

In an effort to put the research findings into practice, we are participating in the training of computer scientists and engineers. This has led to our co-operation with the Department of Computer Sciences at the Swiss Federal Institute of Technology in Zurich.

This report summarises the central findings of the research. In the discussion of alternatives in work design, a series of experiments has produced findings pertinent to the design of dialogue systems. They also point to the significance of the concept of differential work design. By analysing different dialogue structures, a field study illustrated that the dialogue structure itself has a significant effect on whether the user's cognitive control over the computer will be facilitated or rendered more difficult.

The three subsequent contributions are concerned with the organisational use of new technologies. It is shown, for example, that the effects of working with word processors cannot be described globally. Instead, a number of moderating factors have to be taken into consideration.

The introduction of word-processing systems to a federal agency presented an opportunity to redesign work. The various means of carrying this out, as well as some of the problems that occurred, are discussed.

Finally, the setting-up of a computer-aided personnel information system illustrated that while the possibility for choice exists, a socio-technical approach must be taken from the start. Organisational structure must be included at the earliest possible point in the planning stage.

Alternatives in work design

User-oriented dialogue systems

Several experiments have explored the efficiency of individually developed versus prescribed forms of software dialogue. These experiments have shown that the concept of differential work design is applicable to the development of dialogue procedures.

Software design can generally be evaluated on the basis of a variety of criteria, including "transparency" (the clarity and visibility of the work process), consistency, tolerance, compatibility, support, flexibility/ individualisation and participation. Here we will look at the criterion of "flexibility/individualisation", with a particular focus on *dialogue* and *input tools*.

In an experimental study, two groups of women experienced in computer use were presented with different types of dialogue for handling a customer order. Type 1 dialogue was characterised by a high level of rigidity. Type 2 dialogue, in contrast, had a much higher level of flexibility in terms of the user making a choice concerning procedures and multifunctional adaptability of the keyboard.

There was no significant difference in the time taken to perform the task between the two groups. It became apparent, however, that working with the rigid type of dialogue resulted in more significant errors than was the case with the more flexible dialogue.

Further results may be broadly summarised as follows:

- The greater scope of action allowed by the flexible dialogue was utilised by the subjects.
- The increased utilisation of degrees of freedom did not result in additional strain or decreased performance.
- Individualised work procedures stimulated the women to become innovative in that they offered numerous suggestions for improvement.

Another approach to the issues of flexibility and individualisation in computer-aided work activity is illustrated by the study of Ackermann.[2] His approach is based on the concept of differential work design.[3] In order to study the efficiency of individually developed versus prescribed forms of dialogue, Ackermann constructed a computer game in which it was possible to combine single commands into command strings (macro-commands). The subject's task was to steer a robot through a maze to complete a sorting task. The subjects were to perform the task using both individually developed and previously established command sequences. The results of this experiment may be summarised as follows:

- In more than half of all possible comparisons, individually developed command sequences resulted in greater efficiency than preset command sequences.
- Personality differences became apparent in that so-called "situation-oriented" subjects formulated significantly fewer single commands than "action-oriented" subjects and failed to combine them into macro-commands. "Action-oriented" subjects used more freedom in procedure and design of the task than "situation-oriented" subjects did.

Another study dealt with the issues of flexibility and individualisation by looking at input tools.[4] A five-finger mouse[5] with a multifunctional keyboard was designed because it was felt that it might contribute to more efficient dialogue. The experiment used the computer game described above. According to the experimental design, the correspondence between the basic commands of the game and the function keys was either pre-established or chosen by the subjects themselves. As a control, a group of subjects worked only with the usual input medium, the keyboard. The findings to date can be summarised as follows:

- In terms of the relevant parameters for efficiency, the keyboard group showed the poorest results.
- In terms of the relevant parameters for command efficiency and error statistics, individual use of the keys proved superior in a majority of the comparisons.
- Subjects using individually labelled keys made fewer errors as a result of confusing functions than did those using pre-established key-function correspondence.

In each of the experiments described, the findings so far lend support to the relevance of the concept of differential work design for dialogue procedures.

Analysis of dialogue systems

In order to obtain more data on the experience and requirements of computer users in office work, we designed a field study on the basis of previous investigations.[6] Our objective was to compare different forms of VDU work and employee-computer interaction.

Our premise was that the introduction of new technologies is an *option*[7] and that the computer is a useful tool in carrying out work tasks. An important goal, then, is to simplify the tool, at the same time providing a wide variety of possibilities for application. Software adapted to the user's perception, memory, thinking and behaviour is, in this sense, "user-friendly". The user's mental model of the work process and available tools is of central importance.

Two major barriers to effective use of computers are the lack of "transparency" of many dialogues and the insufficient number of possibilities for influencing the sequence of operations.

The field study was conducted in two of the largest insurance companies in Switzerland and in a commercial trading firm. Through interviews and questionnaires, 58 employees of the three companies were asked to judge the quality of the dialogue system they use with respect to several psychological aspects. In addition, the employees were observed while working at their terminals.

The sample consisted of qualified office clerks who had used computers one or more hours daily over an average period of two years. The average age of the employees was 30 years old, and the proportion of female employees, at 38 per cent, was somewhat less than that of males.

Various types of computer systems were found to be in use:

- central mainframe computers with on-line operation to workstations for applications such as bookkeeping and various insurance transactions, and telex and word processing for the specialists;
- word-processing systems (stand-alones);
- decentralised terminals and personal computers (at present used only to a small extent, but increasingly in insurance companies).

There was a general trend towards increasing the automation of work processes and the integration of partial processes, along with slow-moving, step-by-step decentralisation of mechanical storage and processing capacity (networks and multifunctional workstations). Accordingly, greater efforts to standardise and formalise areas of work previously untouched by electronic data processing (EDP) could be expected.

All employees taking part in our study perform demanding and comprehensive work activities within special areas of competence. The manner in which computers are used as an aid in these activities varies greatly.

In the three main departments selected for study, computer systems primarily support the following activities:

Company 1 (insurance): registration and processing of claims; correspondence
Company 2 (insurance): compilation of insurance policy offers; correspondence
Company 3 (trade): registration and processing of orders; correspondence

Figure 1 provides a breakdown of the different categories of computer activity in each of the three companies in relation to the total daily time spent working a visual display unit (VDU). Of particular interest is the relatively high percentage of data-entry time in Companies 1 and 2 in contrast to Company 3, where there is a more balanced relationship between the different categories.

There is also a qualitative difference. In Company 3, computer-aided work is completely integrated into the employee's total activities, while in the other two companies it is an isolated task.

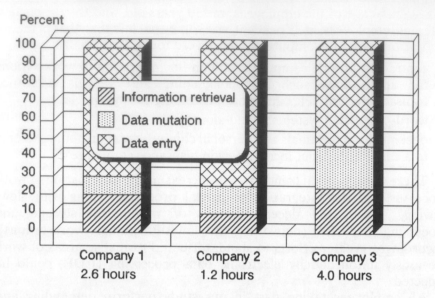

How do the employees rate the support provided by the computer system? In Company 3 we were impressed that the evaluation was completely positive. The benefit to the employees was seen mainly in the simplification and reduction of routine, administrative work ("less paperwork") and in the extensive possibilities for information retrieval. The latter provides enormous support in connection with customer services especially through supplying data on articles (such as inventory, delivery dates, parts replacement, etc.).

Employees in Company 1 also consider the instant accessibility of up-to-date information to be a help, but see this advantage as being offset by the "unpleasant extra work" (e.g. an increase in number of administrative work-steps) required for the registration of damage. The original expectations of these employees of being relieved of routine work were generally not fulfilled. Company 2 takes a middle position in its rating, in that its computer system – particularly in the processing of big jobs – provides assistance by taking over certain routine tasks without adding complications to other work.

When questioned about changes in their work activity since the introduction of dialogue systems, a majority of the employees stated that the work activity had become less difficult, but that the work pace had increased. In addition, pressures to perform, the demands for concentration and accuracy and general job strain had also increased.

These results coincide with the findings of pilot studies, in which employees described work with VDUs as "simpler, yes, but somehow more strenuous".

The exchange of information between user and computer takes place in all three companies by means of a VDU terminal and a keyboard. In each case, dialogue is constructed on basic techniques – menu,[8] data-entry and information "masks" (a format in which data and choices are shown on the screen) which are also known as "passive" dialogue forms. However, the overall structure differs from company to company.

In Company 1, the hierarchical order of the individual elements is arranged according to criteria of both the (mainly mechanical) logic of procedure and the type of insurance. This "mixed strategy" results in a muddled (and thus difficult to retain) overall structure; it also necessitates taking unwieldy "detours" for certain process steps. Obsolete parts of the programme add to the confusion.

The dialogue design in Company 2 was determined by a similar strategy. However, as a result of the company's dealing with only two types of insurance, a consistent set of inter-related menus was developed. In addition, the data-entry masks were placed in a predetermined sequence. This increased automation of the entire work process, made the overall structure of the dialogue simpler, more uniform and more terse.

The dialogue in Company 3 was also designed using a "mixed strategy", but one which clearly differentiates between various parts of the overall structure. Thus, all of the work areas are offered at the first level (main menu), and they can be differentiated at the second level. Plausibly defined processing units which are relatively homogeneous (i.e. self-enclosed) follow. The consistency with which this structure was designed greatly contributes to its terse form.

Dialogue functions in Companies 1 and 2 are limited to those absolutely essential for completion of the task. In contrast, in Company 3 additional helpful functions (such as interruption, sorting, statistics, etc.) are available from the outset. Similarly, the search capabilities available in dialogue 3 through the various possibilities of combination, their broad range of application (customers, objects, orders), and the minimal demands of entry allow the goal to be reached more quickly than in either of the other dialogues.

The system in Company 3 offers the most to the user. He or she can almost always move "forward", "backward" or "sideways" at every level; in addition, by jumping over the second-menu level, the user is able to proceed directly from the main menu to the desired mask. In this regard dialogue 2 stands in sharp contrast to dialogue 3, while dialogue 1 takes a middle position. Dialogue 3 also provides the greatest number of areas of application, as indicated by the number of choices per menu.

As expected, dialogue 3 was, without exception, given a more positive rating by its users than either of the other dialogues. The most pronounced differences related to the dimensions of "flexibility" and "feedback". Thus, objective differences among the dialogue structures in terms of opportunities for personal styles of behaviour are clearly reflected in the user evaluations. The predetermined dialogue path was evaluated negatively by the users in Company 1 and even more so by those in Company 2. In the interviews they described their feeling of being pressed into approaching a task in a certain way, thus being degraded to the role of a servant of the computer ("feeding" data).

The more negative evaluation of "feedback" (in dialogues 1 and 2) can above all be attributed to the fact that, in the case of erroneous data entry, while correction references are provided, the cause of the error is insufficiently, or not at all, explained. Learning processes, essential for the modification and refinement of mental models, are thereby rendered more difficult or even made impossible. Differences among the dialogues with regard to the possibility of forming adequate mental models are not as great as were expected. Apparently, daily use of the computer system enabled users in Company 1 to form in their minds a structural and process model of the dialogue. Differences in the evaluation of "transparency", which refers more to the outer form of dialogue structures than to the facilitation of the forming of mental models of them, are more pronounced. Here the effects of practice play only a subordinate role.

The users of dialogue 1 in particular are forced to retain in the memory too many details which are difficult to differentiate in terms of meaning.

In the overall evaluation, dialogues 1 and 2 do not differ at all. Apparently, the minimal "transparency" and average flexibility of dialogue 1 offset the completely absent flexibility and average transparency of dialogue 2, as far as the ratings are concerned. The extraordinary significance of dialogue flexibility is seen in its high correlation ($r = .70$) with the scale for "evaluation". The greater the flexibility rating of a dialogue by the users, the more positively it will be rated overall.

In sum, a "user-friendly" dialogue system should, according to our subjects, exhibit the following characteristics: broad field of application; user control; use of understandable terms and symbols instead of codes, abbreviations, and so on; uniformity; self-explaining error messages; short response times (about one second); and guarantees against system breakdown. In addition, the desire that programmes be better tested before their release for use and that users be given more opportunity to participate in the process of software development was expressed. In response to a direct question regarding users' preference for a simple, system-guided dialogue versus a more complex one offering more degrees of freedom, we received an impressively clear answer: 84 per cent of those questioned chose the type of dialogue which allows the user to develop individual action strategies, even if mastery of such a tool required the acquisition of a greater amount of knowledge. This can be understood as a sharp rejection of all those concepts in which "user-friendliness" amounts to foolproof, system-guided dialogues, praised for being easily learned and operated.

Concluding remarks. The results of this study confirm the hypothesis that interaction with computers is primarily a problem of "navigation" and only secondarily – at the input/output interface – a problem of communication. The *cognitive control* which the user has over the computer is, according to our data, of decisive importance. The components of this control can be described as possibilities of *orientation* ("transparency", predictability) and of *exerting influence*. Furthermore, it is also important that the system should offer a broad range of possible uses in a task-compatible way. And finally, it seems to make sense to provide opportunities for the individual to make choices – for instance, by providing user-definable keyboard functions.

Alternatives in organisational design

The use of word processors in Switzerland's federal government administration

Switzerland's federal government administration is divided into seven ministries, comprising approximately 85 federal agencies. For this study on the use of word processors in the federal government, 15 federal agencies were selected as representative.

The *employees* were, in addition to managerial staff, academic and technical personnel and task specialists, secretariat employees include secretaries, some having specialist functions; copy typists and clerk typists; and typing supervisors. About 90 per cent had had specific commercial training. Two hundred and thirty-six women employed within the secretariats (84 per cent of all secretaries) took part as subjects. About

22 per cent of the secretariat employees studied were employed on a part-time basis. A hiring freeze ordered by Parliament must be seen as a special condition in this area of work.

Work activities of secretarial employees consisted of: typing; general secretarial duties, such as handling mail, copying, telephoning, filing, and so on; and task-specialist work in different areas of competence.

The secretaries were asked to apportion their total activity in terms of the above components in order to present a clearer picture of their activities. Cluster analysis of the responses resulted in five distinguishable categories of secretarial jobs:

	Type	Number of employees
Type 1	Clerk typists	52 (22.0%)
Type 2	Secretaries	83 (35.2%)
Type 3	All-round secretaries	59 (25.0%)
Type 4	Executive secretaries	21 (8.9%)
Type 5	Task specialists	21 (8.9%)

The average percentage shares of the component tasks in the five categories are shown in figure 2.

Job satisfaction. Ratings of important aspects of the work situation varied greatly and corresponded to the type of job.

The all-round secretaries rated their jobs from good to very good; the secretaries and task specialists rated their jobs as average; and the clerk typists rated their jobs as rather poor.

In addition, the estimation of the employees of their satisfaction with important features of their work situation showed analogous conclusions. In total, the findings point to the importance of an adequate mix of secretarial work activities.

Still, for many employees in the secretariats (of all work types), there is a problem of incongruity between their actual qualifications and the qualifications required for their work activities. This means that not only *could* many of the secretaries studied perform more demanding tasks (on the basis of their training and experience), but they also expressed the *desire* to do so. The opportunity to use one's abilities and knowledge, as well as the opportunity to learn, seem to contribute significantly to the evaluation of job satisfaction.

Chances of promotion for employees of secretariats – almost exclusively women – are rather small. Accordingly, their average satisfaction with "promotional opportunities" was lowest among the categories investigated.

Figure 2 **Work activities of secretarial employees in the Swiss federal administration – as reported by 236 employees in 15 secretariats**

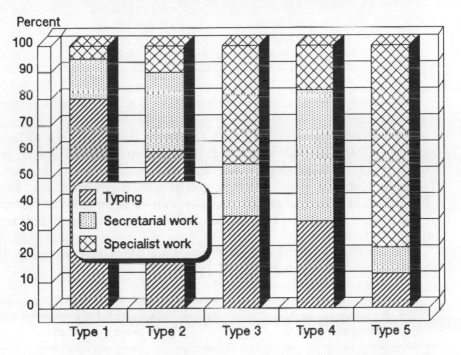

Word processor use. In the 15 federal agencies selected for the study, 41 word-processing systems were in use at the time of our investigation. Of the 236 secretariat employees, 101 (42.8 per cent) used word processors for at least a part of their typing work. The remainder used typewriters exclusively. The percentage of word-processor users ranged from one-sixth to all of the secretariat employees in any given agency.

The average daily amount of time spent working with a word-processing system was reported by the employees as follows:

Amount of daily use	Number of employees
Less than 1 hour	5 (5.4 %)
1 – 1.5 hours	6 (6.5 %)
2 – 2.5 hours	8 (8.6 %)
3 – 3.5 hours	12 (12.9 %)
4 – 4.5 hours	36 (38.7 %)
5 – 5.5 hours	12 (12.9 %)
6 – 6.5 hours	8 (8.6 %)
7 – 7.5 hours	3 (3.2 %)
More than 7.5 hours	3 (3.2 %)

Work with word-processors involves text entry/editing and handling of repeated text.

Written material produced with the word processors, in order of decreasing frequency of occurrence, includes many-paged documents; routine work (with predetermined and standardised text-constructing elements); statistics, tables and lists; and general correspondence. Tasks other than text editing are of the sort that can be designated as "classic" administrative secretarial duties. Such tasks vary greatly in content from one agency to another.

The spectrum of activity of word-processor users differs significantly from secretaries using conventional typewriters:

Proportion of working time spent per day	Typing	Secretarial work	Specialist work
Word-processor users	63.8%	21.3%	14.9%
Non-users	41.9%	29.0%	29.1%

Thus, word-processor users spend a greater amount of their working time typing than their colleagues using conventional typewriters. The reasons for this difference include the fact that word-processor users are often assigned comparatively more typing work and also that newly introduced word-processing systems act as magnets, attracting additional typing tasks. This is, however, not the case in all the agencies. From this, we see that it is possible to use word processors in different ways.

The effects of working with word processors are modified by various factors, including, for example, the way in which processing work is organised, the structure of total work activities, the length of time spent working with the VDU, the type of written material handled, and so on.

With regard to effects on health, it was found that persons using a word processor three or more hours daily estimated the incidence of certain physical complaints to be more frequent than those spending less time working on the VDU. Complaints reported included eye troubles, nervousness and pain in the fingers and/or arms.

Those secretariat employees who were affected by the introduction of word processors were asked about the subsequent changes. The following tendencies were noted:

- The introduction of word processors had mixed effects. While negative aspects such as fatigue, pressures to perform, job strain and work pace increased, certain other effects, such as increased challenge and a slight reduction of monotony, were positive.
- Work with word processors made increased demands on knowledge, abilities, accuracy and, especially, powers of concentration.
- Users report no great change with respect to opportunities for social contact. This is a reflection of the fact that, in the Swiss federal administration, word processors are not being used in highly centralised typing pools.
- There has been practically no increase in the volume of routine work. This may change in the future if, in addition to long documents requiring repeated revisions (the most frequent present use), word processors are also used to handle standardised written texts.
- The most marked effect of word processors concerns the authors of the texts. Authors have tended to take less care in producing draft texts and have increased their demands for correction or revision.

Organisational alternatives in work with word processors. Since the agencies all possess a certain degree of autonomy with regard to organisational issues, a great diversity of organisational structures exists within the secretariats. We found two extremes in secretariat organisation:

Agency 1: Strict separation of typing and administration. In two word-processing secretariats, typing work is done centrally and the remaining administrative jobs are performed in several administrative secretariats. Only the secretaries in the word-processing secretariats use word processors.

Agency 2: A total of eight small secretarial units of two to three employees each. These secretariats perform all duties falling under the subdivisions of the agency. The word processors are at the disposal of all the secretariat employees, although there are capacity problems.

It was found that the differing organisational structures, as well as different ways of structuring activities, are highly significant factors in the way that subjects experience and rate their work situations.

The secretariat employees rated their possibility of participating in decision-making concerning work and organisational structure from "very little" to "very great", depending on their agency. Many of the employees pointed out how important it would be in the introduction and organisation of word-processing work to have direct influence. They believe that this would facilitate the creation of an optimal work situation.

Conclusions and a look ahead. Several effects of the introduction of word processors were identified in this survey. These effects depend on the way systems are put into use, on organisational structures and on the structure of the total work activity, particularly the mixed nature of the activity.

At the onset of our survey (February, 1984), 49 of 84 agencies within Switzerland's federal administration had word processors at their disposal. The first word processors were introduced in 1978. Since then, many more agencies have obtained word processors for their secretariats.

According to current plans, secretarial and task specialist work will eventually be related by means of larger, more integrated systems. It is unclear, however, just when such systems can be introduced. For the time being, word processing will continue to represent the major application of new technologies in the secretarial area.

The increasing integration of new technologies will certainly have more extensive consequences for secretarial work than those found in the present survey. Whether or not these effects will be of a positive or a negative nature will depend to a large extent on how the new systems are organised.

Design attempt I: Secretariats of a federal agency

The following section describes an attempt to use the introduction of word-processing systems as an opportunity to make organisational changes within the secretariats of a federal agency. The project, commissioned by the directors of the agency, contained both rationalisation and humanisation goals. Employees of the secretariats were to participate actively in the process of change.

The project took place within the existing organisational form, and was restricted to traditional work activities in the secretariats. This meant that the goal of designing work adapted to human needs was limited to a reduction of the division of labour *within* a particular section or department. Any changes *among* organisational departments or structures was excluded. To accomplish this, co-operation had to exist between section/department heads and task specialists, who are mostly male, on the one hand, and between section/department heads and secretaries on the other.

The agency is divided into several departments, some of which are in turn divided into sections. Work groups are, as a rule, composed of a section head, task specialists and one or more secretaries. The division of work is characterised by unity of organisation and task. This means that in most cases each autonomous organisational unit works on self-contained task areas.

This results in relatively low dependency on other departments. It is left to the individual units to distribute work among the persons within the unit. Between the departments and sections the division of labour is according to "product", and, apart from central services, there is nearly no division of labour according to task.

Interaction among the departments occurs primarily as a result of dealings with outside institutions, for example when preparing drafts or reports to Parliament. Such matters require co-operation and occasional teamwork. Normally, co-operation between departments occurs solely at the level of the departmental head.

The work activities of the approximately 30 secretaries employed in this agency can generally be classified as "mixed"; that is, they include typing, conventional secretarial tasks (mail, appointments, filing, distribution, etc.) and task-specialist work which varies in scope and quality from area to area. Through an analysis of work activity, it was found that the secretaries spend about one-third of their work time on typing tasks. Their particular mix of tasks approximates the description in the previous section of the "all-round secretary" or "executive secretary".

As a rule, secretaries are directly assigned to department or section heads and thus to a particular task area. As a result, it is possible for the content of task-specialist work and typing work to coincide. Even copy-typing gives the secretary the opportunity and the motivation to learn about the work area, since the content of documents to be typed and the content of specialist tasks are similar or even identical in subject matter.

Implementation of the ideal system. The participation model of the project included the secretaries. They participated through a subjective analysis which allowed them to evaluate their work situation and, from this, to derive suggestions for change including their conception of the ideal way to work with the new systems. On the basis of a questionnaire, a number of features of the work situation were rated according to importance. In addition, the degree of satisfaction with those features was also rated. The questionnaire results served as a basis for later evaluation of changes and were intended to encourage the employees to reflect upon their current work situation.

The results were reported back to the subjects on the same day that the questionnaires were filled out, in order to stimulate in group discussions an evaluation of the existing situation and the development of goals. This method resulted in the cataloguing of desired changes and suggestions for their realisation.

The secretaries primarily criticised the content of their work, finding it unchallenging. They also criticised the limited degree to which their work allowed them to take on responsibility, make use of their abilities and knowledge and increase learning. The most negatively evaluated aspect of work was the limited possibility of promotion and the opportunity to learn. These aspects were closely connected with the aspects of work which were found to be in need of improvement.

Very broad limiting conditions resulted partly from the conceptions of the secretaries of the ideal organisational use of word-processing systems. A set of objectives worked out by an internal project group related primarily to an adherence to "mixed" activity in the secretariats and to an increased delegation of area-specialist tasks to the secretaries. Important objectives were defined as (1) task areas for each co-worker according to her abilities; (2) specialist tasks which comprise task areas as self-contained as possible; and (3) restriction of the time spent typing, in general, and of work with the word-processing system in particular, to at most 50 per cent of daily working time.

As a result of the secretaries' input, it became evident that there was a need to become increasingly involved in the work of the department or section, not only in terms of information but also in terms of the kind of work itself. The secretaries experience their work, on the average, as "reduced to" copy-typing and support functions. They would welcome the addition of more demanding, area-specialist tasks and would be in favour of greater opportunity to participate in other tasks and to increase their learning.

Organisational alternatives: Initial experiences. Overall, an attempt is being made to take advantage of rationalisation gains created by the use of word-processing systems so as to allow the secretaries to take on more task-specialist work. Changes are taking place in different ways, as can be shown in the cases of the following two departments.

In one of the departments, the secretaries' task areas and sphere of duties were revised at an early stage to increase their share of task-specialist work. At the same time, partly new assignments were given to those for whom the secretaries typed in order to create work areas more self-contained in terms of content. The technical-organisational solution chosen was a "technical pool" (a separate room for the word-processing system), with access to the system regulated by the users themselves, according to a rough time schedule.

In another department, a different solution was chosen. Here, additional and more interesting tasks are not distributed equally or similarly among all the secretaries, but are given to only a few persons. One secretary has been promoted to task specialist; her share of typing now corresponds directly with her assigned task area – in other words, she has become her own secretary. Only one or two other secretaries receive a somewhat increased share of task-specialist work, whereas one-half of the secretaries will most probably continue to have the usual "mixed tasks". This sub-group is potentially in danger of experiencing an intensification of workload combined with a lack of diversified, in-between tasks.

Different forms of job enrichment thus become apparent; they differ in the form of distribution of new tasks to co-workers. In certain areas, however, the possibility was never completely ruled out that a secretarial position might be taken over by a half-day typist, who would work more or less exclusively on the word-processing system. This solution resulted in a very non-mixed activity (typing only) for at least this one person. Thus, in addition to the secretaries, there is now a copy-typist – an example of centralisation of operations within departments.

Whatever model of task redistribution is put into practice, the changes should have the common result of triggering something which affects co-operation within the sections or departments – that is, there will be a change in co-operation and in the division of labour between superiors and task specialists on the one hand, and between superiors and secretaries increasingly entrusted with area-specialist tasks on the other.

One of the most significant aspects of this project is the fact that the authorities in charge of technological innovations had stipulated that word-processing systems be distributed relatively sparingly and be employed to capacity. In some federal agencies, this resulted in the setting up of central word-processing pools and, thus, to the demotion of secretaries to typists. This centralisation of operations can be seen as the consequence of giving higher priority to the optimal use of technology than to a meaningful use of human resources.

For administrative work the question arises as to the extent to which traditional forms of the division of labour could be surmounted through the advanced utilisation of EDP methods – for instance, through having workstations totally equipped with personal computers or EDP terminals. However, the application of technology on a large scale could result either in minimising the differences between the activities of task specialists and secretaries or in intensifying the division of labour within an organisation.

Design attempt II: Personnel administration in private industry

The following describes a project in the central personnel division of a multinational firm based in Switzerland. The firm was about to modernise its technically outdated personnel information system. We were asked to use this revision of the system as an opportunity to improve the organisational structure within the company, by means of a participative design model.[9]

As initially designed, the project's proposed changes were far-reaching. Although technically possible, they only became a reality in part. It became apparent that certain mechanisms can hinder the optimal design of the organisation-technology interface.

More than 200 persons are employed in the company's central personnel division. Four sub-departments were studied:

- two sub-departments within the Department of Personnel Services, each employing seven secretaries (with commercial education) and six task specialists (with commercial or university education); and
- two sub-departments within the Department of Personnel Administration: "Personnel data", employing seven task specialists (mainly trained on the job, with a few having commercial education), and "Salaries and Wages", employing eight task specialists (the majority having commercial education and a few trained on the job).

Up to the summer of 1985, all four sub-departments used a personnel information system based on batch processing. In 1981, the personnel division requested the EDP department to develop an alternative to this system which handled 120 different business events and data on over 40,000 persons. Since the summer of 1985, approximately 80 end-users have been at work on 44 VDUs linked on-line to a central mainframe computer. Most of the terminals are shared by two employees (involving no shift work).

In administrative areas the system is mainly used for the input and processing of data; in the area of personnel services its main use is for data entry and retrieval. The proportion of time spent working at the terminal varies from employee to employee. Normally not more than a third of total working time is spent at the terminal; as a rule, this is not a block of time but is spread over the total working period. This is mainly because work at the terminal is almost always coupled with task components not requiring the terminal. Typical monthly fluctuations in terms of workload can be controlled by the employees, as the system allows data entry in advance.

The software design meets most of the criteria for user-oriented dialogue systems. Nevertheless, most of the work activities could not be judged humane in the sense of the definition given in the introduction; this is primarily due to the extensive division of labour. Although the affected employees had expressed their needs and made suggestions, the technical innovation was not accompanied by organisational and structural innovation. When designing work organisation, however, there exists a critical moment of decision affecting the quality of jobs.

Work and task organisation in the Department of Personnel Administration. The centralised Department of Personnel Administration maintains certain kinds of information on employees. The administrative work is divided into six task areas: personnel data, salaries and wages, management systems, credits, expenses for personnel and data processing. (Other personnel responsibilities, such as recruitment, development and personnel services, are assigned to other departments.)

The sub-department which handles personnel data is further divided into units handling data on work attendance, general and skills data and code systems. Within the unit concerned with attendance, the task areas are handled by one employee who processes data on absenteeism and two employees who process shiftwork and overtime data. Within the unit handling general data and skills data, the various tasks are handled by one employee who processes data on skills; a second who processes general data; and a third who processes problem cases encountered by the first two employees.

As can be seen from the above examples, each employee is working in a very limited task area. Co-operation among the employees is not necessary. Neither at the level of the individual employee nor at the level of the sub-department is there a unity of product and organisation. Co-operation is required, however, with employees of other sub-departments, as when, for example, reports of overtime work lead to changes in wages. The interdependence of tasks here can be designated as "isolatedly independent".[10]

The work activities examined here are characterised by a high degree of repetitiveness and low cognitive requirements. Typical monthly fluctuations in the amount of work result from batch processing. A qualitative lack of challenge is therefore coupled at times with a quantitative overload. Job content is evaluated negatively by a majority of the employees; they expressed a desire for increased variety, greater challenge, more opportunity to learn and increased opportunities for co-operation.

Organisational alternatives and impediments to realisation. The technology of the personnel information system is flexible to a degree that would allow the building of very diverse organisational structures. It would be possible, for example, to integrate previously isolated task areas so as to make the division of tasks less extreme. With the employees, we evaluated the work situation and discussed ideas for possible new work structures.

Three types of change in organisational structure could be carried out:
- integration of tasks within the unit;
- integration of the task of "Personnel Data" and "Salaries and Wages" (these sub-departments show a similar division of labour); and
- integration of the tasks of the "Personnel Administration" and "Personnel Services" departments.

In each of the above cases, the quality of work activity would be improved. We believe, however, that only the second and, in particular, the third variants would result in decisive improvement. Here the forming of partly autonomous work groups would be possible and expedient.

Discussion of the latter two variants met with considerable resistance. Their realisation would have required the dissolution of existing organisational structures and the setting-up of new ones; upper management declared that such changes would not be feasible. The first variant is at present being put into practice; this will lead to various kinds of job enrichment for individual persons and small groups within the sub-departments. The main impediment to further improvements will be organisational and political principles which may not be challenged. The cause is not to be found (or, at most, to a very limited extent) in technological restraints.

There is a significant danger that the organisational principles required during the stage of centralised data processing will continue to be followed, even though the necessity for them no longer exists. The question is whether this occurs because of a lack of insight into the disadvantages of such forms of organisation or a lack of perception of the options presented by *interactive* systems, or because of the advantages that these forms of organisation bring to the holders of certain positions in the organisational hierarchy.

Most often, the reasons that technically available options are not used are to be found not among the technicians and EDP specialists but rather among those who commission the EDP projects. This fact comes into view at an early stage. First, issues of work organisation are scarcely or not at all recognised as possible goals of the projects; and secondly, the organisation of the projects (that is, positions of responsibility, procedures, planning, forms of user participation, and so on) is often unilaterally determined by EDP concerns. There may be a third factor in that certain already established units of the organisation may engage EDP specialists in their own interest and may thus commission the development of a system which will fit the already existing form of organisation.

Work systems that are developed primarily for partial units of an organisation do not necessarily represent the best solution for the entire organisation. However, a comprehensive, all-encompassing approach can also meet with difficulties. Proposals for changing existing structures can, or even must, lead to opposition, because they threaten to affect the established structure of power.

It has become clear that organisational restrictions originally arising from technological limitations can gain their own independent existence, insofar as they hinder the creation of more imaginative solutions which new technologies make possible. Restrictions today, however, result from organisational rigidity in holding on to existing organisational structures.

Consequences. When new technologies are applied to work and organisation in terms of individual jobs alone (and/or only with regard to organisational units which are isolated from one another), there is a danger that less than optimal results will be achieved. This is true not only with regard to designing work that is adapted to human needs, but also in relation to the technical possibilities. A socio-technical approach that deals with larger organisational areas than the units analysed and restructured is needed from the beginning. The potential of the new technologies can be utilised only when existing organisational structures are not seen as unchangeable limits. If a socio-technical approach can be taken, this can lead to a hitherto uncommon alliance between scientists of work and organisation on the one hand, and EDP experts on the other. Such an alliance would offer promising prospects for both groups: technology could be implemented in the service of employees while, at the same time, technological possibilities could be exploited to achieve more highly integrated and humane applications.

Office of the future: Trends and premises**

Through our study of the "office of the future", we hope to be able to answer the following questions concerning the future development of office work:

- What technological changes can be expected within the next ten to 15 years in office work?
- What skills will be required of employees as a consequence of these changes?
- What changes in organisational structure and what options in organisational design can be expected?
- Are there widespread chances for electronic work at home?
- What kind of vocational training is required to cope with the changed demands?
- During what period will these changes occur, and to what extent?
- What will be the consequences for the labour market?

These questions relate to three main topic areas: (1) work content, skill requirements and educational demands of the office of the future; (2) period and extent of the changes; and (3) consequences for the labour market.

Plan of research

Hypothetical models for each of the three main topic areas were developed through interviews with experts from companies using computers and with computer manufacturers and a survey of the literature. In each of these models, those variables assumed to have implications for the above areas are represented. Examples of such variables include technology, performance and function of future office equipment, organisational structures within companies, infrastructure and cost of utilisation of public networks, occupational categories in the field of office work, feasibility of the implementation of new technologies in small and medium businesses, general economic trends, participation of affected employees in the implementation of new office technologies and cost of future office-work systems. Our goal is to acquire knowledge on the variables themselves, the weight of their influence and the extent of their mutual dependence in relation to the three topic areas.

In the first area, for example, we plan to determine the extent to which the quality of work in the office of the future will depend on organisational concepts, and the way in which future office technologies could best be implemented with regard to the adaptation of work and organisation to human needs and qualifications. For this, it will be necessary to determine the interactive effects of future office technologies and organisational concepts within companies. A significant question will be the extent to which future change will affect the various occupational categories including whether or not occupational segmentation will continue to be necessary.

Some premises regarding the future of office work

At present one of the goals of technological development is the integration of all relevant functions of office automation into a single, multifunctional workstation. A great many of the requisite functions are known today, and some, such as telecopying, are already operational. Some are already under development, such as expert systems to support management staff, teleconferencing capabilities and technical means of producing written text on the basis of spoken text. The use of multi-functional workstations will make sense only when the technological requirements of efficient digitalisation of images and speech and the installation of high-capacity public networks with optical fiber technology have been met.

Future office employees will probably use complex technical devices and previously unfamiliar forms of communication. They will increasingly have to deal with more abstract material, and there will be a reduction in simple routine tasks. Work processes will be formalised and regulated to a greater degree, and social isolation on the job could increase as it becomes possible to perform all tasks at a multifunctional workstation.

The manner in which the new office technologies will be organisationally embedded will have a great influence on future office work. In our view, technology is an option: this means that it can be put to use in very diverse ways for various purposes. The way in which technology is used will determine the psycho-social consequences for the affected individuals. This may be clearly illustrated with electronic work at home. When this work takes place within the home of the employee, the consequences could be negative (social isolation, the intermingling of work and home life, etc.). However, if we are dealing with neighbourhood centres or satellite offices, in which several jobs are set up together, these disadvantages could possibly disappear, and the advantages of not having to commute and of reintegrating living areas and workplace could become apparent.

Technology is only one of the factors influencing the development of office work, but clearly one of the most important. By using technology in a particular way, office work can be shaped and designed. Whether or not the possibility of using technology to benefit men and women is realised, however, remains largely a political question.

Notes

* In this report, the introduction and the section on design attempt II were contributed by Christoph Baitsch, that on user-oriented dialogue systems by Eberhard Ulich, that on analysis of dialogue systems by Philipp Spinas, that on the use of word processors in the federal administration by Luzian Ruch, that on design attempt I by Norbert Troy, and that on the office of the future by Christian Katz.

** At the time of writing, this research project can be described only briefly, as it has not yet been completed. The discussion is limited to hypotheses and premises.

1 E. Ulich: "Vorwort des Herausgebers", in J. Linke: "Determinanten und Konsequenzen des Führungsverhaltens in industriellen Arbeitsstrucktruen", in E. Ulich, (ed.): *Schriften zur Arbeitspsychologie* (Bern, Huber), Band 36, 1982, pp. 5-7. This definition was subsequently adopted by the Swiss National Research Program 15, "Arbeitswelt: Humanisierung und technologische Entwicklung" [The work environment: Humanisation and technological development].

2 D. Ackermann: *A pilot study of the effects of individualisation in man-computer interaction*, Proceedings of the 2nd IFAC/IFIP/IFORS/IEA Conference on Analysis, Design and Evaluation of Man-Machine Systems (London, Pergamon, 1985).

3 E. Ulich: "Ueber das Prinzip der differentiellen Arbeitsgestaltung", in *Organisation Industrielle*, 1978, No. 47, pp. 566-568.

4 D. Ackermann; J. Nievergelt: "Die Füng-Finger-Maus: eine Fall-studie zur Synthese von Hardware, Software und Psychologie", in H.J. Bullinger (ed.): *Berichte* des German Chaptger of the ACM (Stuttgart, Teuber, 1985).

5 A mouse is the term for a small, hand-held, movable device which is used in conjunction with a computer terminal to point to specific areas of the display screen to carry out functions. Its introduction by several manufacturers is an attempt to reduce the dependence on keyboards and to make microcomputers more "user friendly".

6 P. Spinas: *Bildschirmeinsatz und psycho-soziale Folegen für die Beschäftigten*, Bericht über die 26, Sektion Arbeits- und Betriebspsychologie im Berufsverband Deutscher Psychologen, Fachtagung Fortbildung in der Bundesrepublik Deutschland (Duisburg), 1984, pp. 367-384.

7 E. Ulich: "Psychologische Aspekte der Arbeit mit elektronischen Datenverarbeitungs-systemen", in *Schweizeriche Technische Zeitschrift*, 1980, No. 2, pp. 10-15.

8 "Menu" is a term used for a collection of items, for example a list of the contents of a system pertaining to a given parameter (directory or file) from which the operator may select.

9 E. Ulich: "Subjektive Tätigkeitsanalyse als Voraussetzung autonomieorienterter Arbeitsgestaltung", in F. Frei and E. Ulich (eds.): Beiträge zur psychologischer Arbeitsanalyse, *Schrifter zur Arbeitspsychologie*, Number 31, (Bern, Huber, 1981), pp. 327-347; C. Baitsch and F. Frei: "A case study of worker participation: Some suppositions, results and pitfalls", in H.W. Hendrick and O. Brown, Jr. (eds.): *Human factors in organisational design and management* (Amsterdam, Elsevier/North Holland, 1984), pp. 385-393; W. Duell and F. Frei (eds.): "Arbeits-Mitarbeiter beterlingen: Eine Heuristik qualifizierender Arbeitsgestaltung", in *Schriftereihe Humanisierung der Arbeitslekens*, Vol. 77, (Frankfurt, Campus, 1986).

10 G. Susman: *Autonomy at work: A sociotechnical analysis of participative management* (New York, Praeger, 1976).

4 New technologies in banking, retailing and health services: the British case

R. LOVERIDGE, J. CHILD AND J. HARVEY *

Introduction

In the United Kingdom, as in other advanced industrial countries, the shift in employment since the 1950s from manufacturing and primary industry into direct services has been significant enough for the term "post-industrial age" to be frequently applied. In 1955 manufacturing accounted for 40 per cent of employees in employment; in 1984, 26 per cent. Meanwhile, the service sector has grown from 45 per cent to 65 per cent of the employed workforce. The sectoral shift has been accompanied by an occupational shift. Within the manufacturing industry, according to 1985 figures from the Department of Employment, a much higher proportion of people are in non-manual occupations, particularly scientific, technological and professional ones. Yet the optimistic belief that service employment would compensate for the loss of manufacturing jobs has yet to be realised, as has the hope that a general upgrading of knowledge and skills would follow from entry into a post-industrial age.[1]

The reasons are manifold but generally derive from the manner in which such forecasts were made. They were little more than crude extrapolations from the structures of employment within firms that existed 20 years ago. It was supposed that the rates of growth among administrative, professional and technical workers would continue to increase exponentially while reductions in manual occupations would steadily decline. The collapse of traditional areas of employment in the manufacturing sector has combined with rationalisation in service industries to produce the type of short-term changes illustrated in figure 1. This illustrates not only the dramatic nature of the decline in craft and operator jobs, but also the reduction in junior office work formerly done by full-time women workers and in managerial jobs previously occupied by men. The expansion of the service sector has taken place as a result of increased productivity, as well as by an increase in the number of full-time jobs created. This has been

Figure 1. Occupational distribution and change by sex, 1981-83

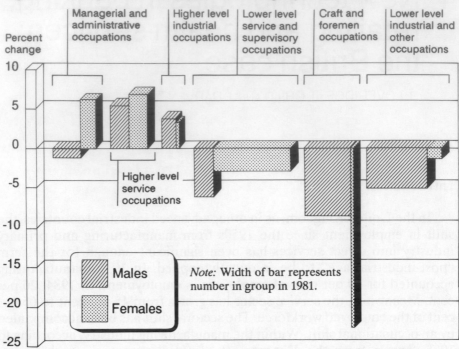

Source: Manpower Services Commission: *Labour Market Quarterly Report* (May 1985).

due not only to greater investment in new technology, but also to an increase in the marginalisation of work. In the service sector part-time and casual labour has long been a significant proportion of the workforce, and women in particular have been seen by potential employers to be especially suited to these types of work. Virtually all women's manual work in the public sector is on a part-time basis. Over the last decade, part-time employment has attracted increasing numbers of women into the active labour force. If current trends continue, nearly half the workforce of the the service sector will be women by 1990, and half the jobs they occupy will be part time. They are heavily concentrated in sex-segregated occupations and are employed at levels of pay and with statutory rights and benefits that are significantly lower than those for men.[2]

One of the purposes of this study was to discover the effects of new technology on the structure and conditions of employment at the point of service delivery. The pessimistic view of the impact of new technology was expressed by Marx in 1867[3] and later by Braverman in 1974.[4] The competitive drive towards rationalisation would cause innovation to take the form of deskilling and restructuring work. Taken together with the social marginalisation of job-holders, this might lead to a flexible workforce but with workers unable to participate in the control of the workplace, or even their own careers.

The pessimistic view of innovation also sees this malleable workforce becoming increasingly isolated from control over capital since the expropriation of their knowledge goes hand in hand with the concentration of ownership and centralisation of organisational management. By contrast, the optimistic view sees the application of information technology as enabling greater participation by workers and consumers in the planning and delivery of services.[5]

The authors have taken the pragmatic view that the direction of change would be heavily influenced by the existing distribution of power in the labour market and the degree to which groups of employees were able to influence the adoption of new technology within their own place of work. The employment areas chosen for study were selected with a view to analysing the effect of worker participation through unions or professional associations on technological innovation. In hospitals 90 per cent of the staff were members of trade unions and professional associations. In banking, the proportion was much less (about 60 per cent) and with many more in employer-sponsored staff unions. In retailing, the figure plummets to around 25 per cent, with a high level of self-employment and casual work. The labour market also represents varying degrees of closure of entrance to new recruits. Whereas in hospitals this control was jointly regulated by staff and management with professional associations playing a dominant role, in banks and in retailing the internal labour market was dominated by the employer.

In this paper each of these sectors are examined in turn. In each case the relative impact of electronic data processing (EDP) on front-office and back-office task is examined. "Front office" means the point at which a service is offered to the client or customer in the first instance. In hospitals this is the reception, diagnosis and treatment of patients. We have been mainly concerned with patient information systems and the provision of intensive-care nursing. In personal banking this concerns cash withdrawals, credit deposits and advice on account management. In retailing it is the registering of cash transactions at the point of sale.

"Back office" tasks largely involve the provision of services to the front-office operator together with the systematic processing and analysis of the data from front-office transactions. In banks and retailing it involves taking a balance of transactions and controlling stocks and flows of cash and commodities through cheques, giro (post office) transfers, bills of credit, invoices and receipts. In hospitals it involves the provision of paramedical services (such as pathological laboratory tests) and records of patient movement.

Health care in the United Kingdom

The National Health Service (NHS) is now the single largest employer of labour in the United Kingdom; it is also the largest enterprise in Western Europe. Its employees cover all occupational grades. Concerned as it is with socialised medicine, it is the second largest item of public expenditure after national defence. Presently, it is constrained by spending limits and government-inspired changes in structure designed to promote greater accountability and efficiency. The necessity to stay within the bounds of nationally prescribed cash limits has led to a shedding of direct labour and a move to external subcontracting of many manual services and some professional ones.

The development of new technology and policy surrounding its implementation must be seen within this context. It must also be seen in relation to the competing identities and uneasy alliances between the various professional and quasi-professional groups whose cross-cutting interests add to the complexity of health care management. Rivalries exist, too, between different levels of the managerial structure and between the many different trade unions concerned with representing NHS workers. In all of these arenas, ethics, moral precepts and patient rights are debated and brought to bear on issues concerning new technology.

The application of new technology within health care has always been incremental, halting and piecemeal. The formulation of a computing policy for the NHS has become a contentious issue in itself. Investment in new technology appears to have been relatively low; a spokesperson from the Department of Health and Social Security (DHSS) estimated it at half of 1 per cent[6] of annual expenditure on health care. Nevertheless, it is seen to have added significantly to the cost-inflation spiral of health services.

The Korner Report (1982) and the Griffiths Report (1983) carry considerable implications for new technology and should provide a framework for technology applications as a management tool to create a more efficient, responsive and accountable health service.

80

Main characteristics of the health sector

The NHS was created in 1948. It was to replace the previous mixture of private medicine and charity, to encompass a comprehensive range of care and to be universally available on the basis of need.

The system that emerged gave considerable autonomy and resources to general practitioners, but ensured that hospitals remained the chief focal point, since in the United Kingdom these also provide education and training for all medical and paramedical employees.

NHS expenditure has been slowly rising in real terms since 1948, despite the fact that the United Kingdom spends a significantly smaller proportion of its national income on health care than do its Western counterparts. In the first year of its creation, the NHS cost 79 pounds sterling per capita of the population. By 1981 this had risen to 240 pounds sterling per capita (adjusted for inflation).[7]

This increase is in part symptomatic of demographic changes resulting from an ageing population. For example, in 1951 the population aged 65 years and over numbered 5.3 million. By 1982 this group had risen to 8.1 million. The number of people surviving to at least age 75 rose 26 per cent between 1975 and 1985. The demands for health provision that this figure represents are compounded by the fact that the cost of servicing an individual's health needs accelerates with age.

Rising costs have led to efforts to account for this trend, such as shorter hospital stays, together with increased centralisation of control and the use of management techniques mentioned earlier. There has also been an increasing concern to address a pattern of disease which has shifted away from acute illness towards the chronic problems of the aged, requiring an emphasis on care rather than cure.

Over this period the number of people employed in the Health Service has also increased, from 400,000 in 1949 to double that figure in the 1980s, that is 825,800 full-time health workers. Seventy-five per cent of NHS workers are women, making the NHS the largest employer of women in the country. Women workers in the sector are predominantly employed as nurses or ancillary staff; the more senior and well-paid occupations are generally male-dominated. In contrast to the expansion in staff, some contraction in plant and equipment has taken place since 1979, with the closing of 90 hospitals and a loss of some 13,000 beds.

While implementing a policy of fiscal stringencies in the public health sector, the Government has sought to promote private health care facilities, for example in tax relief to companies to cover their contribution to employee subscriptions and the relaxation of restrictions on private hospital development. In tandem the Government has directed hospital

81

management to shed labour in certain areas of hospital employment such as laundries, cleaning, catering and maintenance in favour of privately subcontracted labour.

The development of technology policy in the National Health Service

The system of capital procurement in the National Health Service (NHS) allows a wide spectrum of interests to participate in the allocation of resources. Overall cash limits are set by Parliament and specific constraints by the Department of Health and Social Security (DHSS). Below that level, specific allocations to management boards at regional, district and hospital level are based on a bidding system in which specialist departments vie with general administrators to make a case for specific budget allocations each year. Technological innovation has generally proceeded by means of initiatives by heads of departments (normally physicians or surgeons) and in a largely incremental fashion.

The potential uses of computer technology within the NHS were acknowledged during the late 1960s. Several computer projects were established in England and Wales under the auspices of a DHSS experimental research and development programme responsible for investigating computer applications in different aspects of health care. Other projects set up at the time were financed from regional or individual hospital funds. By the mid-1970s only 20 hospitals in the United Kingdom were using their own computers and these had largely been financed under the DHSS experimental scheme. They were devoted to administrative systems such as records of patients, waiting lists, bed allocations and a master patient index. By late 1977, the DHSS programme had succeeded in creating a number of good working systems but had failed to produce a standardised model.

The programme had in fact encouraged a diversity of approaches in order to derive a number of options for use throughout the service. The move towards what Illich has described as industrialised medicine[8] was given further impetus by the 1974 NHS reorganisation which sought to rationalise and unify the organisational structure of the service while promoting a new managerial approach to health provision. The DHSS produced successive reports in 1973 and 1974 – *Review of NHS computing* – on the then "state of the art" in health service computing. Other systems in existence in the early 1970s were based on large batch-processing mainframe computers at regional headquarters providing a region-wide bureau service in most parts of the NHS. These were largely confined to such data as payroll processing, accounting and child health administration. Clinical applications such as whole body scanners and the monitoring of the vital signs of patients had been taken up to some extent, but with considerable regional variation. Such medical innovations were pressed through the highly fragmented and political system of bidding for resources and therefore appeared in a somewhat random fashion.

The late 1970s saw a shift in government health concerns. The 1976 report on *Priorities in health and personal social services in England* contained a critical appraisal of the cost effectiveness of high-technology medicine combined with an assertion that medical resources must be diverted towards the improvement of primary care (defined to include community care in addition to general practitioners). In many ways this was an attempt to claw back resources from powerful medical consultants who had been successful in obtaining investment for the treatment of acute illness, and to redirect resources towards the elderly, the disabled, the mentally ill and children. The approach was coupled with an emphasis on preventive medicine and health education. Many authors have argued that this is a matter of economic expediency more than a principled stance against "industrialised medicine". Significantly, the report argued: "preventive medicine and health education are particularly important when resources are tightly limited, as they can often lead to savings in resources in other areas".

Following in the wake of this, the DHSS experimental programme was finally discontinued in the late 1970s. Computer developments were felt to have become commonplace, an ordinary administrative expenditure. This, coupled with problems of implementation outlined in the 1973-74 computing reports, put the responsibility for investment onto the regions.

Health authorities now make their own decisions concerning electronic data-processing equipment, and it is they who must decide how much they are willing to spend on this area from their general funding allocation. Centrally funded technological initiatives are now confined to small-scale, pioneering computer applications, such as computer-aided diagnosis.

At the same time, falling hardware costs and the advent and growth of minicomputers served to stimulate EDP in hospitals. In 1981 a survey of all 199 districts revealed that 87 per cent of respondents had access to a microcomputer, and overall, 302 microcomputers were in use.[9] They were utilised for a variety of functions from clinical work to finance, building maintenance and personnel files.

Shortly afterwards, in late 1981, a further attempt to avoid organisational duplication of effort and to monitor advantageous developments was made. A NHS policy committee was appointed and charged with ensuring cost effectiveness in relation to information technology. (At the same time, regional computer policy plans were to be drawn up. Many regions failed to comply, and this notion failed). The committee was considered to be regionally dominated, and has since been superceded (in 1984) by the central Information Advisory Group, on which there is greater district representation.

This development is linked very closely to the recommendations of the Griffiths Report.[10] Griffiths maintained that: the "NHS Management Board should cover all central aspects of NHS management, including Health Authorities and non-departmental bodies. It should control directly the work of the Supply Council of the NHS Training Authority together with the work of computer policy and health information, since at present their position in the NHS executive management line is not clear." The brief of the newly created Information Advisory Group is therefore to advise the NHS Management Board on central computer policy in the light of local needs.

The return to central direction in purchasing computers coincides with Griffiths' objective to identify and activate management roles and increase accountability and feedback of needs throughout the system. Information technology is therefore seen as an indispensable tool for management and management education. Griffiths' wish to further involve clinicians in management, particularly in the sphere of budgeting, may also carry implications for innovation in administrative systems, since consultants are among the chief disseminators of technology in clinical uses.

In pointing to these needs, Griffiths serves to underline and agree with the concerns of the Korner Committee[11], which sought to provide the means of compiling essential statistics systematically as a basis for rational decision-making and improved managerial control. Korner recommended that the service should aim to provide integrated patient information, requiring an integrated patient administration system. Specifications were given for a minimum data set for a patient information system and for the compilation of a data base covering the use of NHS facilities.

The adoption of EDP in hospitals has been beset with difficulties relating to user education and local conditions for implementation. Indubitably these have constrained progress, but other more strategic factors have also intervened. In particular, the structure of decision-making and the relationship between medical and administrative needs as expressed within that structure have played a major part in fragmenting effort and diffusing direction.

Industrial relations

Coincidental with the establishment of the NHS, a hierarchy of management-union negotiating bodies was established. These were based on the so-called Whitley principles in which no clear distinction was made between matters of joint consultation and those of bargaining. Of the nine councils established, seven represented medical or paramedical groups, one administrative staff and one manual staff. A General Council brought together representatives from all bodies at the national level, but in no hospital was an attempt made to activate the formal provisions for a joint staff council. In addition to their union representation, most professional groups participate in the management of the NHS through specialised "teams" and in the setting of standards for their work and responsibilities to patients.

Unionisation among manual and paramedical staff remained low until the 1970s. Work relationships were largely paternalistic with a high degree of shared trust between levels of well-marked hierarchy. Cash limits placed on NHS spending in the 1970s combined with the effects of reorganisation on local relationships to create a climate in which these relationships changed dramatically. Membership of trade unions affiliated with the Trade Union Congress rose from 18 per cent to 66 per cent in the decade before 1979. At first union action was focused on pay rises, later on opposition to closures and redundancies.

The unions have paid little attention to the effects of new technology other than the joint monitoring of health and safety implications of its use. The main administrative and clerical union, the National Association of Local Government Officers, has been successful in negotiating upgradings for word-processor operators, and new technology agreements have been implemented in some authorities. Our study has revealed many instances of clerical staff, nurses, paramedical and medical staff undertaking new tasks in the areas of programming and systems maintenance with no significant change in pay or status. Unions have made no inroads into the design stage of technological innovation, and consultation prior to the installation of new technological devices has been limited to exchanges couched in terms of managerial prerogatives. Development of a coherent union strategy has been inhibited by the incremental nature of most technical change. Succeeding generations of machines have been introduced with additional functions that have remained unscrutinised by the unions. Practical negotiating difficulties arise, too, because of the consultants' practice of bypassing the NHS funding structure and buying equipment with charitable donations. Such acquisitions circumvent the usual funding procedure and are difficult to hinder, particularly in light of the shared adherence of unions to an ideology of enhanced patient care.

The range of technology

Technology within the Health Service falls into two broad categories: information technology used for processing patient and management data, and clinical applications which may be of a diagnostic, physiological monitoring or analytical nature.

In terms of information technology used for processing patient and management data, the most salient to the central workflow of the hospital is the patient administration system. Patient administration systems can cover, for example, the filing and retrieval of medical records; computer-based nursing treatment records (including the planning of nursing care); drug prescription and drug interaction programmes, which provide information to prevent patients from receiving inappropriate, inaccurate or potentially dangerous combinations of drugs; bed allocation facilities and occupancy records for beds and wards; and scheduling and results of routine tests.

From this index, appropriate statistics can be extracted and analysed. All wards and departments can be networked to the system via visual display units (VDUs), and can thereby have the facility to call up or input information at will.

More developed patient administration systems may also encompass facilities for arranging appointments and recall of patients, the scheduling of clinics, management information systems, and hospital organisation and administrative data. Other systems have been developed to cover most areas of medical specialisation, community health care and epidemiology as well as accountancy and the control of stocks and flows of resources.

Clinical applications are equally various and complex. First, there is the imaging technology, including gamma cameras, ultrasonic scanners and whole body scanners. These new non-invasive techniques have enabled more accurate, more detailed, less dangerous and less painful patient investigations, often on an out-patient basis. Another area that is developing is that of computer-aided medical diagnosis. Applicability is limited to areas of medical diagnosis where only a limited range of readily cited and quantifiable symptoms exist, and where their underlying causes are relatively well associated. In such cases, computer diagnosis is as accurate and more procedurally consistent than diagnosis by most doctors.[12]

86

Microprocessors in general practice are now also coming into fairly general use. These may in principle take the form of patient medical record systems or may be concerned with personal history-taking either directly from the patient or via an intermediary. (Computer-aided diagnosis and computerised drug-interaction programmes would also be applicable in this field.)

Computerised analytical equipment

Biochemical laboratories test samples of blood, urine and other body fluids for evidence of a number of pathologically derived systems. This is done by mixing the samples with appropriate chemicals and physically shaking them or submitting them to centrifugal forces which separate out the molecular constituents in an analysable form. The shaking was formerly done mechanically, while the testing involved the manual insertion of instruments into a multiplicity of test tubes.

Virtually all biochemistry laboratories now have 70 to 80 per cent of their test load on one machine, i.e. some form of auto-analyser. Auto-analysers were developed in the 1960s and initially (and to the present day, in many cases) they were based on the continuous flow principle. Some of the later machines have been centrifugal analysers. Auto analyser development has now reached the fourth generation and most NHS laboratories will possess either a fourth or third-generation machine. Under the earlier technologies, results were printed out by the machine in the form of graphs. These had to be calculated and interpreted by technicians and the results had to be manually transcribed. At the end of the day, technicians had to come together to collate their results with those obtained on other tests for the individual patient. Auto-analysers can obviate this process by providing a complete profile of one or several specimens which have been submitted to a battery of tests. These will then be transmitted on-line to a computer which will print out the results. (There is presently some debate over whether such machines produce too much data, with some laboratories choosing single-test or discrete-testing machines.)

One of the earlier claims for automated laboratory machines was that they would release technicians for more interesting research work. Despite a reduction in the clerical functions of technicians, this prediction has not been fulfilled, since the introduction of such machines has been accompanied by a vast increase in the workload. The scientific, craft-based skill of manual chemistry and graph reading has become the technical skill of scanning large batches of numbers and error messages. The fear expressed by some technicians was that they would become machine operators. Despite their claim to a job rooted in a knowledge of clinical chemistry which facilitated accurate quality control in the automated context, they almost invariably felt, nevertheless, that auto-analysers had served to deskill their work.

Details of particular technical tasks will vary according to whether the analyser is based on the continuous flow principle or that of centrifugal force, but at the analysis stage the technician will basically be engaged in feeding the machine and monitoring the analysis process. On the basis of this monitoring and the results produced, the technician must then decide whether or not to accept the result generated or re-run the particular sample. The exercise of this discretion will require reference to such factors as control samples, risk of contamination from a previous sample and whether the machine is in phase with the rate at which the samples have been passed through it.

The results are then read automatically and recorded through a computer print-out. The lab technician must then scan these results for abnormalities. "Every test is different, but the basic movements are the same," lamented one technician. Increases in test numbers ranging from 100 per cent to 250 per cent over a ten-year period have been recorded in laboratories, without concomitant increases in staffing. The role of central (district or hospital) laboratories is now threatened by the spread of miniature analysers being used by physicians to conduct their own blood gas tests in the wards. These might remove some routine tests from laboratories while leaving more comprehensive or specialised tests to be done centrally. Techniques are also under development which would permit biochemistry to be conducted by means of non-invasive techniques where testing is carried out on the patient's skin surface without the requirement of drawing off blood or fluid.

At present the effect of automatic analysis on the hierarchy of tasks in the laboratory appears to have removed much of the skill and knowledge contained in the three years of education required for the technician (Medical Laboratory Scientific Officer – MLSO) quali-fication. It has, however, created the need for new skills in accessing and programming the data files maintained on computer within all the laboratories we observed and with its use in trend analysis. This work has usually evolved to senior technicians who create their new roles with no formal national acknowledgement of the change.

All of the initiative for the introduction of auto-analysers has remained with laboratory heads. These are often medical doctors, but the position has increasingly become occupied by a natural scientist (biochemist). The deskilling of technician jobs reinforces the duality of the market structure in laboratories, a duality which can be seen to follow gender lines. The possibility of increasing polarisation of tasks and rewards towards a core and peripheral divide appears to be emerging. Trends indicate that the MLSOs carrying out the remaining 25 to 30 per cent of non-fully automated work will all be graduates (the number of graduates recruited with this type of work has been rising steadily over the last few years), while the routine automated tests will be carried out either by non-graduate MLSOs or possibly laboratory aid staff. In either of the latter cases the suggestion is that such tests will be covered by female staff since the majority of non-graduates and laboratory aid staff are likely to be female. This would not represent a discontinuity from the current situation since the majority of women MLSOs work below the supervisory level where the routine testing is conducted. A senior MLSO is the first level entailing supervision.[13]

The new automated technology, operating alongside a management ideology which informally resists investing promotional prospects in female staff, could result in the formalising of this already observable sexual division of labour in the laboratory. This would become especially salient should the task of operating an auto-analyser be broken away from its professional moorings, since its level of routinisation is readily co-existent with such conditions of employment as part-time work, low pay and the formation of an occupationa l cul-de-sac in career terms. All these characteristics are stereotypically associated with "female work".

This would largely represent an extension of the current situation in the United Kingdom, where, although a career hierarchy exists, case study material suggests that female MLSOs generally do not receive encouragement to participate fully in training and promotion opportunities or to get involved in work experience increasingly associated with positive promotion prospects and upskilling, such as data processing. In the United Kingdom, the higher the hierarchical position amongst MLSOs, the fewer the number of female staff. Heads of laboratories are reluctant to invest promotion opportunities in women who they assume will leave employment to have children and rear them. This becomes part of a complex self-fulfilling prophesy, where, with a lack of hierarchical female role models, a discriminatory environment and a lack of alternative childcare arrangements, female MLSOs do indeed leave employment, often to be recruited later in life to part-time, dead-end jobs within the same service or even the same laboratory.[14]

Intensive care units arose from the need to bring together nursing and medical expertise to support patients with multiple medical problems. The strategy became possible because of technological developments, such as lung ventilators, the refining and extension of anaesthetic techniques and the development of close monitoring techniques. Nurses in this area receive additional training in understanding the physiological changes associated with critically ill patients and instruction in the use of monitoring and respiratory equipment. The nurse must call for the assistance of a physician or anaesthetist should the patient's condition deteriorate beyond certain predetermined limits.

Patient monitoring. The vital functions that are typically monitored include heart rate, pulse rate, blood pressure and central venous pressures. Trends and cross-comparisons produced by recording such measures allow anticipation and swift intervention in deteriorating situations. These readings were, and to a large extent still are, taken by hand and visually. The connection of body nodes to a bedside display unit or instrument panel is also normal practice. The introduction of microcomputers enables the readings to be recorded, analysed and displayed on video monitor in a more sophisticated way than could ever be possible using paper and pen. In some ITUs (intensive therapy units), monitors may be connected to central nursing stations or they may be on-line to patient data handling computers. The organisation of observational care in this way is potentially labour-saving.

In the United States a further refinement has taken place. Under certain conditions the monitoring technology "closes the loop" and, having monitored the patient's vital signs, proceeds to carry out self-correcting action by the administration of a drug, should the computer programme suggest this to be necessary. Such devices could arguably lead to an erosion of nursing and medical expertise and discretion. British doctors represented within our research were unanimously opposed to closed-loop systems.

Our study indicated a strong commitment to the philosophy of bedside nursing, regardless of the details of the technology adopted. This commitment was reflected throughout the different levels of nursing and medical hierarchy. The nurses welcomed video monitors as useful aids, but saw them as complementing rather than replacing their more direct patient observations, such as noting the patient's complexion and respiratory state. Electronic blood pressure monitoring via the use of transducers appeared to be a contentious area, and fears of inaccurate reading frequently led nurses to often doublecheck or bypass such technology and resort to the manual technique of taking the pressure "on the cuff". There was some evidence that use of the technology was a factor in dissuading nurses from entering ITU nursing.

Patient data information system. One ITU within our sample had installed a computerised patient data information system. There are still relatively few of these in Britain. Interconnected terminals and video screens were situated at the bedsides of patients, in nearby operating theatres and in the biochemistry laboratory. Data input was primarily carried out at the bedside of patients. The histories of patients were integrated with body readings. It has been estimated that more than 500 values each day can be generated by an ITU patient, and the computer was seen as an accurate and rapid means of processing this output. Doctors generally valued the system and consulted it frequently. Time was saved by avoiding paper handling, and a full and accurate, easily accessible record was afforded. Nurses were divided over the extent to which they found the computer of use. Approximately half of the nurses questioned felt that little advantage was gained either in terms of time-saving or creating a more accessible form of data. They also felt the actual data collected supported the medical role of the doctor rather than the care role of the nurse. Keying in data at the bedside, coinciding closely with the predominant and pervasive bedside ideology of the unit was, however, welcomed by all, and the computer link to the biochemistry laboratory had come to be seen as essential. As a byproduct of the keyboard system, the nurses often had acquired typing skills, and it was suggested that some nurses were thus prepared to record far more free-text comments than they would under a manual recording system.

Nurses in intensive care units derive an unusual amount of authority from their one-to-one close observation and care of the patient and their familiarity with complex medical cases, when communicating with doctors. The ability of doctors to consult the computer did not appear to undermine the position of nurses in this respect. The doctor still had to seek amplification of points from the nurse, and the doctor would still need to inform the nurse of any change in the patient's treatment. Invariably, too, the initiative to alert the doctor remained with the nurse, who would usually be the first person to see any results or observe significant changes in the condition of the patient.

Ethics and control in the National Health Service

Medical technology raises a number of ethical and moral issues not raised by many other technologies, since it intervenes in the provision of care and the prolongation and saving of life itself. It affects the very epidemiology of mortality, morbidity and disability. It is a contentious area in that some have argued that medical technology appears to have added years to ailing rather than healthy lives.

Technology, such as life support systems, has also served to place the medical profession in situations where they must increasingly decide how long to maintain positive technological intervention when the possibilities of survival are minimal. Confidentiality is also a major issue – that is, who has access to particular information and on what basis? Many argue, in fact, that security risks are lessened by computerisation, but the bringing together of personal data on individual patients to which access may be obtained via an interlinked network of terminals must raise public doubts.

In a climate of financial stringency the dominance of the medical profession is under challenge from the growing influence of full-time administrators. The recent appointment of chief executives at national, regional and district levels indicates a move to centralised control in which the influence of the medical consultant is likely to suffer. So far the influence of new technology has been a counterbalancing influence between the centralisation and decentralisation of control in the NHS. Doctors have exercised considerable autonomy in the acquisition and use of microcomputers and electronic machines for treatment or diagnosis. Administrative uses of computers have often strengthened central control through the extended use of existing mainframes.

The present trend, promoted by Korner, is towards the standardisation and rationalisation of computer applications that will undoubtedly aid centralising forces.

Overall, groups that have relied on the power of ethical judgement and deployment of esoteric knowledge are likely to lose position as a result of the widespread introduction of EDP. It is difficult to suggest that the polarisation of work seen in the pathological laboratories will be universal in the NHS. Rather, it seems likely that much of the routine work developed in the use of computer-aided administration, diagnosis and treatment will be sloughed off by the higher professions and devolve to junior grades of staff.

If, however, the sense of professionalism is lost in a new atmosphere of scientific management, lower grades of staff may have more difficulty in retaining their present standing within the NHS.

The banking sector

Increasing competition in banking

The domestic banking system in the United Kingdom is narrowly defined and concentrated in comparison with that of other countries. The largest banks in the retail market are the "Big Four" among the London clearing banks: Barclays, Lloyds, Midland and National Westminster. These banks emerged from amalgamations of city and localised country banks, and have inherited large branch structures giving wide coverage within England and Wales. The Trustee Savings Bank and Royal Bank of Scotland Groups, having recently had internal amalgamations, are now medium to large in size, leaving four smaller banks to complete the domestic sector.

The boundaries between banks and other financial institutions are rapidly eroding. Banks now face considerable competition for personal deposits from the building societies. These societies are sources of private house finance springing from the friendly society savings movement which in countries such as the Federal Republic of Germany, Sweden and the United States became the basis for a large part of conventional banking activities. In the United Kingdom, the Trustee Saving Banks, Yorkshire Bank and Co-operative Bank developed from similar roots among the working class. The lifting of regulatory restrictions in 1980 gave banks the opportunity to compete directly with building societies in loans for house purchase and improvement. The building societies are now awaiting government legislation which will enable them, in turn, to offer many banking services including agency services, securities services and unsecured personal lending. Building societies already hold a larger share of personal deposits than do banks, and the government's national savings schemes have also eroded the banks' share of personal deposits.

Moreover, there has been an increase in competition among banks themselves. Smaller banks offering free banking and an emphasis on personal service have been capturing customers from the Big Four, forcing the latter to do likewise, starting with the Midland in 1984. Among foreign entrants to the industry, American Citibank is planning a major assault on the British market with nation-wide coverage. The chairman of one of the Big Four recently stated: "We could be represented today as being a high-risk, falling-margin industry beset by competition on all sides".[15]

Banks have a prominent institutional role in society, linked to public confidence in their soundness and orderly administration. During the first half of this century they experienced a long period of stability. These two factors encouraged the development of a strong welfare-paternalistic tradition and clearly defined job statuses within almost self-contained, internal labour markets.

All banks operate elongated hierarchical grading (managerial) segments. Except for certain specialist staff in short supply and part-time employees, recruitment is confined to the secondary or tertiary education-leaving stage. Subsequent promotion has depended on the securing of banking qualifications combined with internal managerial assessment. The banks have operated an informal, no-poaching agreement which has inhibited the development of an external labour market. In return, staff have been offered benefits which compare well with other sectors. Employees have had the prospect of internal promotion to appointed grades where pay is relatively generous – a prospect effectively open to men rather than women because it has depended on encouragement to take banking examinations and on a willingness to be geographically mobile. Job security has been sustained not only by tradition but also by a long period of almost continuous growth in jobs. Thus employment in the banking and bill-discounting sector in the United Kingdom rose from 183,000 in 1960 to 385,000 in 1984.[16] There are also substantial fringe benefits including low-cost mortgages and good welfare facilities. Employers also have endeavoured to reinforce staff by funding glossy house journals, clubs and ceremonials.

The Big Four, in particular, have also supported staff associations as an attempt to discourage the intrusion of an external trade union. Three of them still have staff unions, now affiliated to the Clearing Bank Union (CBU), thus dividing staff representation between these and the independent industry-wide Banking, Insurance and Finance Union (BIFU). In the Midland Bank, staff representation is also divided – between BIFU and ASTMS (Association of Scientific, Technical and Managerial Staffs). The CBU has a stronger representation than BIFU among male and higher grade staff – the categories less immediately vulnerable to new technology. Its policy on new technology has been more accommodating to managerial prerogatives, and managements in the banks concerned have taken advantage of this contrast and division between the unions.[17] Of all the British banks, only the Co-operative and Trustee Savings Banks have acknowledged new technology as a subject for agreement with unions.

94

The introduction of new technology by banks has been aimed at reducing the volume of paperwork and growth of staff during a period of steadily increasing levels of business and, more recently, at the qualitative improvement of services and management information. Two overlapping phases in the development of electronic banking technologies have been identified, the first oriented to the centre and the second to the branches.[18]

The first phase occurred mainly during the 1960s. Investment in centrally located mainframe computers permitted the centralisation of customer accounts which had previously been administered by the branches at which accounts were held. The new centralised systems used batch processing, and initially involved transmission of substantial volumes of paper between branches and processing centres. The computerisation of current accounts within the clearing banks in turn facilitated the creation of a system for transferring funds between them by exchanging magnetic tapes. In 1984 an automated inter-bank system was introduced to speed up the clearing of large amounts. While about 80 per cent of all inter-bank and inter-branch clearings still involve the transmission of paper, the automated proportion is steadily rising and, together with branch automation, is restraining the rise in staff. Total clearing volumes rose by 91.5 per cent between 1972 and 1981, while staff employed by the clearing banks rose by only 28.6 per cent over the same period.[19]

The second phase of technological development, the introduction of new technologies into branches, commenced in the early 1970s. Branches were equipped with terminals connected to the bank's computer system. Most of the clearing banks introduced "back-office" terminals which allowed the entry of data into bank networks at the point of origin and also provided an on-line, interrogative facility. Smaller banks concentrated their investment on "front-office" counter terminals which capture data and make account information available to the cashier at the time of the customer's transaction. Counter terminals offer a particularly favourable reduction in the amount of routine branch clerical work. The four main clearing banks are currently experimenting with the use of counter terminals, but British banks as a whole have a much higher ratio of back-office to front-office terminals than do those in other major European countries.[20]

A growing number of customer-operated terminals have also been installed in or outside branches. The intention has been to relieve pressure on counter staff, to displace costs at the counter, to reduce queuing at

95

counters, to avoid expensive expansions or changes of premises and, in the case of automated teller machines (ATMs) located outside the branch or in separate lobbies, to offer an extended-hours cash service. The introduction of external ATMs was initially encouraged by the general cessation of Saturday openings in 1969 and has more recently been stimulated by competition with the building societies which have longer opening hours. By June 1984 there were 6,106 ATMs in service, of which 4,536 were "through the wall", 1,187 were inside branches and 217 were in special lobbies.[21]

A third phase of retail banking automation is anticipated by the late 1980s, involving electronic funds transfer at the point of sale (EFT/POS) and truncation. Both these developments offer the substitution of electronic instructions for the paper instruction of a cheque or a credit card voucher. They could replace large volumes of clerical labour and pose a threat to a high proportion of clerical bank employees in branches and in central clearing departments. Another development may be home banking, though opinion is divided over its likely popular appeal.

Finally, most banks are now developing systems to provide management information, particularly at branch level. These include the computerisation of customer-based files intended to provide information in readily accessed form, suitable for managerial marketing initiatives as well as to save file space.

Bank policies on technology and employment

The policies now being pursued by British banks on technology and employment have to be understood in terms of (1) their forward thinking on service provision and modes of service delivery; (2) the relative influence on this thinking of their technical and marketing functions; and (3) the branch structures they have inherited. These policies are formulated centrally, with little effective influence exercised by banking unions and indeed minimal participation by branch managers and staff.[22] Although there are differences between all banks, it is useful to distinguish broadly between the four main clearing banks and most of the others.

The Big Four banks serve a wide variety of customers ranging from large international corporations, medium-sized companies and local authorities, small business and professional offices down to the private customer who can in turn be differentiated by socio-economic status. The private retail customer primarily requires a money storage and transmission service, including provision of cheque books, information on his or her balance and periodic statements. This customer may, more occasionally, require a loan or an insurance policy, and work may be required in connection with securities. Corporate services are typically much more extensive. In recent years, the large banks have become much more aware of this segmentation of their markets, which leads to a questioning of the traditional assumption that all branches should normally be capable of offering a full range of services rather than concentrating on a particular market segment.

Two other factors are the large branch networks these banks have inherited, which are increasingly expensive to run, and the availability of technology which can automate basic services without apparently eliciting significant objections from most customers. The large banks are therefore tending to move towards branch rationalisation programmes which distinguish between branches offering basic money services and those offering a range of other services including advisory ones. It is technically feasible to provide all the money services automatically through customer-activated terminals, in the lobbies of banks or via external ATMs. Reliance on automation could prove to be an economically attractive solution for urban branches whose customers can readily travel to a "town centre" branch when they require access to non-routine or personal services. Several banks are experimenting with money service automation in those branches which are now open on Saturday mornings, while continuing personal service for inquiries, new accounts and marketing initiatives. The banking unions have expressed alarm that this automation represents the prototype for future lower-tier branches and a serious threat to clerical employment.[23]

The relatively early entry of the clearing banks into mainframe computing, followed by their development of large internal networks, was accompanied by the growth of well-resourced and influential management services (i.e. technical, systems and organisation and management) departments. Our own studies indicate strong belief among the staff in automated modes of service delivery and internal data handling. There is, however, a growing marketing voice counterposed to the advocates of technology. Some have doubts about the cost-saving claims which were made for automation, such as the saving of counter staff through provision of ATMs.[24] Others, wishing to respond to competitive pressures to extend bank services in the retail market beyond low-margin money services, favour the retention of personal staff contact with the customer, and indeed an enhancement of their roles, in order to be in a favourable position to market these additional services. Although we found that personnel specialists in these banks would also wish to influence branch systems policies in the direction of enhanced job content, their role is effectively confined to facilitating staff acceptance of policies decided by others. Their own marginality to the decision process reinforces their position as a buffer between the bank and the unions, in which they serve to keep union representatives at arm's length from any negotiation on the subject of new technology.

The smaller banks, by contrast, are expanding their branch networks, or at least have no plans for closures. Their business is heavily centred on the personal retail market, and the logic of market segmentation does not, therefore, apply to the same degree. Their marketing appeal stresses a personal service to the customer and sympathetic attention to his or her requirements. Their growth makes it easier to absorb technological development and productivity improvement without the prospect of redundancies, which the four main banks are now having to contemplate. Encouraged by the cushion which this growth has provided and, perhaps, influenced culturally by their origins as repositories for working class savings, the Co-operative, TSB and Yorkshire Banks have entered into much closer discussions with the union (BIFU) over new technology developments.

Differences are therefore to be found between banks in their predicted future levels of employment and in their envisaged content of branch services and of work roles within these. There are considerable uncertainties over the returns to be expected from technological developments, partly due to the difficulties in predicting moves by competitors and to the unknown response of the public to future technologies. In these circumstances the large banks are continuing to experiment with a range of branch technologies and to sustain a debate between conflicting strategic considerations.[25] The issue of whether new technologies are used to narrow jobs or to enhance them also remains open. It will depend on the criteria applied to the provision of service to the customer, illustrated shortly. It may also vary with the way in which a tiering of branches is achieved, since this could enhance the role of senior clerical staff if they were given charge of lower-tier branches offering highly automated standard services only. Similarly, changes in the employment of branch managers and loans officers will depend on how a computer-based technique such as credit-scoring is applied.

It is, nevertheless, possible to identify certain trends in banking employment which are connected with sector-wide patterns, such as product diversification and growing competitive pressures, which in turn influence the use of new technologies. These trends are now summarised before illustrating the specific impact of new technologies on the content of work.

Employment trends

There has been an underlying trend of growth in banking employment, but this has been slowing down. According to figures from the Department of Employment, the annual average employment growth increased by 3.5 per cent between 1961 and 1970; by 3.3 per cent between 1971 and 1980; and by 2.0 per cent between 1981 and 1984.

Forecasts presented by Rajan[26] suggest an average annual increase in overall banking employment of between 1 and 2 per cent between 1983 and 1987. Of this increase, about two-thirds is expected to occur in the clearing banks and one-quarter to consist of part-time staff. These forecasts are based on three assumptions, namely (1) a continued increase in the volume of banking business, albeit at a slower rate due to competitive pressures; (2) an increase in staff productivity due to the rationalisation of branch networks; and (3) the confinement of new technology applications to ATMs and counter terminals rather than entry into the anticipated third phase of truncation and EFT/POS. It is now unlikely that substantial progress into this third phase will be achieved during the forecast period. In fact, two expected pieces of government legislation could have an earlier impact on employment through their, respectively, negative and positive impact on business volumes. The first will permit building societies to offer an extended range of banking services, and the second will abolish the right to receive income in cash rather than have it paid directly into an account.

One large clearing bank which expects growth in branch employment of 2 per cent annually estimates that this growth would have reached 3.8 per cent without the continued introduction of new technology. The present wave of investment in new technology at the branch level is primarily directed at reducing clerical and counter work. Counter terminals can offer significant savings in the clerical workload. One of the smaller banks we studied calculates that the installation of counter terminals and related system changes has provided workload savings in branches of about 12 per cent. Employment in this bank has been growing at about 3.5 per cent annually, and the productivity increase can, therefore, be readily absorbed.

Should the large clearing banks adopt counter terminals in large numbers and achieve comparable productivity increases, they would find it more difficult to avoid clerical redundancies. The installation of ATMs so far has not reduced transactions over the counter on the one-to-one basis originally expected. One large clearing bank has found that 2.3 transactions are required via ATMs to save the cost of one transaction over the counter. The number of counter transactions in another large bank clearly fell for the first time only in 1984, once it had installed over 1,400 ATMs. Willman and Cowan's study of a non-clearing bank suggests that installation of on-line counter terminals saved substantially more jobs than did ATMs.[27]

Rajan's questionnaire survey of banks revealed that in a large majority of them, new technology was seen to have reduced clerical employment between 1978 and 1981, though it is not clear how much of this should be attributed to head office and branch reorganisations. Increases were recorded during the same period in other employment categories, namely (1) managerial, professional and administrative, (2) computer-related and (3) advertising, marketing and sales. Some clerical staff appear to have been redeployed into other groups and others redesignated as computer-related when they became involved in keyboard terminal activities. Rajan's respondents nearly all predicted clerical job losses under conditions of static business volumes.

Divergent trends in numbers employed are therefore evident as between those engaged in routine branch clerical and counter work and those in management, specialist services, marketing and computing. The impact of technology is apparent, though it is neither straightforward nor particularly meaningful to disentangle this from branch rationalisation programmes or from the drive to diversify into new services, some of which, such as credit cards, ATMs and corporate cash management systems, would not have been possible without new technology. The divergent employment projections on the whole differentiate those engaged in routine work from those with less routine or specialist activities. This segmentation is also reflected in a growing polarisation of career opportunities and levels of intrinsic job content.

Recruitment, training and career opportunities

A combination of factors is working towards a fundamental change in the recruitment, training and career systems within banks. New technologies have contributed to a growing product sophistication, as in corporate software services and information services in the personal sector. Marketing initiatives will become increasingly informed by customer information systems. At the same time, technology has been used to simplify tasks such as branch paper-processing, till balancing and cash dispensing. Senior bank executives now more frequently articulate a need to recruit high-grade specialists from outside banking to support new and more sophisticated services and their back-up systems, rather than continuing to rely on people who have progressed upwards within the bank.

100

On the other hand, a shift towards recruiting part-time staff to perform branch tasks which have now been simplified is also evident. For instance, during 1984, full-time employment in the London clearing banks fell by 300 while the numbers of part-time (female) staff rose by 600.[28] Part-time staff has increased from 7 per cent of all bank employees in 1974 to 9 per cent in 1984. The attraction of hiring part-time staff lies not only in their lower labour costs but in two other considerations as well: (1) the fact that marginal labour savings from new technology installations in the branches often amount to less than one full-time employee; and (2) part-time staff offers flexibility should it be decided in the future to rationalise branch structures. At both upper and lower ends of the career hierarchy, the traditionally watertight, single-entry internal labour market is becoming more permeable.

In consistency with this policy, the banks have now moved to a tiered system of recruitment. Those recruited on the traditional school-leaving basis at age 16 with four "O"-level passes are now not expected to progress beyond clerical grades. A higher recruitment tier with expectations of enhanced career progression draws on graduates and school-leavers with "A"-level passes. A yet higher point of entry has already emerged for systems and data-processing specialists servicing the development of new technological systems, and is soon expected to extend to proven experts in areas of service diversification.

The tiering of recruitment and career opportunities is likely to reinforce the gender division of labour which typifies banks and which has attracted considerable criticism.[29] This point is illustrated by recruitment figures for one of the largest British banks recently which demonstrates how proportionately fewer women are represented in the higher educational bands.

Entry qualification (Degree/professional qualification)	Male (%)	Female (%)	M/F ratio
2 "A"-level passes	27	8	3.4:1
4 or more "O"-level passes	61	58	1.1:1
Fewer than 4 "O"-level passes	12	34	0.4:1

In the past, career progression depended on Institute of Banking (IOB) qualifications, performance in the job and sponsorship by branch managers which included encouragement to study for the IOB exams. This system worked heavily in favour of male staff and was accompanied by a traditional set of expectations to this effect. It is now acknowledged as an issue by many senior bank managers who do not, however, anticipate any significant improvement. Wastage figures for women who are recruited through the higher accelerated route continue to run significantly above those for men, to judge by figures from one large clearing bank, which cites domestic and family considerations as the main reason for this. Moreover, the steady introduction of keyboard-activated technologies to routine clerical tasks is tending to tie female staff to such tasks because of the male management claim that this is work to which they are better "suited" than men.[30] Hence, female bank employees tend not to be encouraged to progress above clerical grades even though more are now staying on beyond the mid-20s when most used to leave. They are largely concentrated within those very areas of routine branch and central clearing office work that are most threatened by the future extension of new technology in the forms of truncation, EFT/POS, home banking and substitution of manned lower-level branches by unmanned automated lobbies and terminals.

This polarisation within internal labour markets, whereby increasingly distinct skill-cum-gender groups are emerging, has already generated a view within the sector that the traditional IOB certification system is obsolete in at least two respects. First, what is now said to be required for clerical staff is a basic level of training, sufficient for their limited role and which does not raise false expectations that they will progress to holding positions of responsibility as "bankers".

This training would be distinguished from that offered to career staff. Second, the present content of IOB courses is said to be over-oriented to a traditional concept of the branch manager with a strong emphasis on securities and insufficient in areas such as marketing and new financial services.

Impact of new technologies on the content and subjective work experience

The detailed picture that emerges from close investigation serves to qualify any simple view of the impact of new technologies. First, in both banks studied (a large clearing bank and a regional bank), the introduction of equipment to branches was determined centrally, as were the operating systems and associated tasks. Even so, the allocation of tasks to jobs (i.e. to particular employee positions) could vary between branches at the discretion of local management. There is clearly the potential to modify work organisation at this level around a given set of systems and technologies.

Second, the branch technologies impinge to varying extents upon the various tasks performed within the branch. They affect the "back-office" machine room and counter clerks quite significantly, securities staff less so and mainly through receipt of printed information, and managerial staff as yet least of all.

Third, the same hardware such as counter terminals can be configured and programmed so as to perform different functions, and the content of staff roles can be defined with a corresponding flexibility of choice.

Fourth, the general criteria that were in practice passed down from the centre contrasted somewhat in the two banks, and arose primarily from each management's strategy of service provision. These were not technologically determined, but rather influenced the way technology was applied to the organisation of work. The clearing bank was moving towards a differentiation of branch technological and organisational models as its thinking developed on market segmentation and branch rationalisation, whereas the regional bank operated in what it regarded as an unsegmented market and offered a fairly standard package of services.

Thus, while both banks had invested in counter terminals, these were standard equipment in the regional bank but were of varied configuration and still partly experimental in the clearing bank. In the regional bank, counter terminals were introduced to reduce the clerical workload by eliminating recording of transactions on paper, to provide a better service to customers by furnishing more information and reducing waiting times, to increase control over customer irregularities and to avoid the costs of premises by increasing throughput and saving on filing and staff space. The clearing bank has introduced two main counter terminal applications. The first bears some similarity to that in the regional bank, except that the customer is obliged to enter a Personal Identification Number (PIN) via a simple keyboard. This system was introduced by the central technical department without any appreciable consultation and has met with customer and staff resistance. In the second application, staff use the counter terminal to drive a cash dispenser in open-plan units where their roles are restricted to this operation and to providing balance information. The prime objective of both applications in the clearing bank was to speed up counter transactions and reduce queuing times. The support the technology gives in the open-plan branches also served the objectives of improving the bank's customer image, of separating routine cash transactions from others, and of locking cashiers into a time routine under management control.

The consequences of these different ways of using counter terminals for job content and subjective experiences of the staff are summarised in figure 2. The figures indicate that:

- similar equipment can be used to support different work systems and work organisation;
- job content does not change along single trajectories of upskilling and deskilling, nor along those of enhanced or diminished control. The policies pursued in the clearing bank tend towards a greater amount of deskilling and restriction of discretion than in the regional bank. In the latter case, however, some skills such as balancing were no longer required, though other possibly more challenging ones involving relations with the customer were added. While counter staff could exercise greater discretion under the new scheme, and both they staff in the machine room were relieved of pressures, the system gave management more information which it could use for control purposes;
- different categories of staff do not necessarily experience new technology and associated changes in the same way. This was found to apply to full-time versus part-time staff and male versus female staff.

The thinking of banks around counter terminals is not confined to workload savings, nor to speeding counter transactions, but includes the aim of shifting staff from the back office as paperwork and the repetition of data entry is avoided. There may be a saving in numbers, but it is envisaged that other staff will move into direct contact with the customer and engage in the marketing of services. This would add a new dimension to clerical skills which at present is normally recognised by a higher grading. Such a development would almost certainly be welcomed by the staff concerned. One purpose of installing ATMs and other customer-activated terminals is to achieve a similar shift of staff effort towards the generation of new business.

Employment in the back-office machine room is threatened by the third phase of technological development which will involve entry of data at the point of transaction (counter, shop check-out, ATM) and then its automatic manipulation within and between bank computer networks. Our comparisons between on-line and batch-processing machine rooms indicated a clear staff preference for the technological advance to an on-line mode. Working with on-line terminals enabled staff to control the organisation of their work so as, for example, to decide when to deal with intermittent entries like amendments and requests. They also appreciated having the opportunity to exercise skills such as terminal operation. Staff

Bank

Bank	Job content	Subjective experience of staff

Regional bank

Counter terminals operated by cashier only. Used for credits and debits. Account profile appears on screen and cashier can make informed decisions about withdrawals. System automatically balances. Terminals are on-line.

Clearing bank

System 1. Similar to regional bank, except customer has to enter PIN, and VDU does not give full customer profile. Terminals are not used to deal with enquiries.

System 2. Used for credits and debits. Drives automatic cash dispenser. Will not dispense more than £200. Balance information via microfiche.

Job content

Cashiers. Main task lost is manual balancing. System "guides" user through routines. Identification of cashier errors now easier. Cashier has more information on customer, can control illegitimate withdrawals, and can more readily contribute to cross-selling.

Machine-room staff. Reduction in work load and back office work easier to keep up-to-date. For all staff: less pressure of work at end of the day.

Similar to above, except system limited to cash transactions and additional effort required to ensure customers enter PIN.

Counter role narrowed down to cash operations and balance enquiries. Considerable pressure to maximise speed of transactions. Cashier responsible for discrepancies but does not balance own till.

Subjective experience of staff

Part-time staff report they now have less freedom to choose their own method of working and less knowledge of how well they have done their work. Male staff tended to see counter terminal system as diminishing the skill and responsibility previously associated with cashier work. However, the majority of staff (full-time female) experienced no deskilling and welcome loss of routine paperwork as well as the ability to finish work earlier. Their main irritation is when a systems failure occurs.

General dislike because the system is not seen to bring any significant advantages. Customer reluctance to use the system places an additional pressure upon staff and creates dissatisfaction.

Full-time staff dislike narrowing of role (deskilling) and management pressure to increase transaction speeds. Part-time staff welcome simplicity of the role and avoidance of complications such as till balancing.

Figure 2 Summary of changes to job content and to subjective work experience following the introduction of counter terminals in two banks

working in machine rooms where work is batched up and sent to a local data-processing unit did not regularly use a terminal. Those who had previously worked with an on-line system described a sense of deskilling, and job dissatisfaction has also been reported among those employed in the data-processing units.[31]

Currently some banks arey developing branch information systems based on customer data captured when accounts are opened and through subsequent updates. These systems are intended to enhance the marketing role of managers and senior branch staff, though within a context in which more rigorous evaluations of branch performance are being imposed.

The possibility that credit-scoring techniques based on customer files will replace the personal judgement of managers and loan officers over the approval of lending bites deep into their traditional roles.[32] The combination of these techniques with the downgrading of branches under rationalisation schemes threatens to remove some local managerial employment and to deskill the jobs of others down to the mere supervision of residual clerical duties.[33]

Future developments

The potential lines of future technological development in banking are already discernible. These lie in the further substitution of paper records and communication by electronic technology; in the extension of systems integration both within the banking sector and outwards to embrace other financial transactions including retailing; and in the continued development of information services for customers and the banks' own managements. The employment implications of these trends add up to a massive replacement of clerical labour and the growing importance of systems specialists and of staff who provide the professional input for information services.

What actually transpires will depend primarily on the policies of service provision which banks adopt in response to competitive forces and with technological possibilities in mind. The inability of banking unions to influence such policies appears likely to continue unless involuntary redundancies were to generate a mobilisation of active member support.[34] The issues of consequence include (1) how fast and far banks will diversify into relatively labour-intensive areas of business such as insurance, securities brokerage, travel, estate agency and mortgages; (2) whether there will be a significant rise in the percentage of the population possessing bank accounts; (3) how rapidly and extensively banks will move into truncation, EFT/POS and home banking; and (4) what branch concept(s) banks will adopt.

Branch concepts revolve around different modes of service delivery. Hedberg and Mehlmann have constructed five possible scenarios of Swedish bank branches in 1990.[35] The main dimensions concern (1) the degree of automation of cash transactions, arrangement of small loans, account information and provision of general financial information – within branches, in separate lobbies or in the home via interactive viewdata; (2) the emphasis placed on personal advisory services and marketing for deposits, loans and other services; and (3) the range of non-traditional services provided in the branch. At one extreme, branches could be transformed into completely automated service stations. Alternatively, they could combine automation of routine transactions with advice-giving and marketing on a personal, friendly, open-plan basis, or they could deploy a range of technology-based and personalised services in a boutique mode.

The last option, of extending the range of branch services, offers the best prospects for maintaining employment levels and injecting additional skill requirements into bank jobs, but it is difficult to tell how profitable and competitive such branches would be. Large branches providing a wide range of retail and corporate services would require higher-level specialist and managerial skills. Small branches confined to routine transactions and aided by automation may require no more than supervision by someone in a higher clerical grade. The decision on how far to automate the loan-granting process also bears on the branch managerial role and has not been finally resolved in most banks. Even within an unchanged branch structure, the development of in-house information systems around customer details plus the more ample provision of terminals opens up the job design options. The decision has to be made as to whether to use the technology to inform and enhance the jobs of staff dealing directly with customers, or to reduce their discretion through a precisely programmed definition of questions to be asked, steps to be followed and responses to give.[36]

New technology in British retailing

Trends in retailing

The retail industry is one of the most significant employers in the United Kingdom. In 1984 it constituted some 10 per cent of the employed labour force and was the largest area of employment for part-time workers, casual workers and self-employed workers. Overall sales volumes increased by nearly 59 per cent (at 1978 prices) between 1960 and 1982. Yet the value of retail sales actually decreased as a proportion of personal disposable income, from 53 per cent in 1950 to only 39 per cent in 1984. This is largely explained by a shift in consumer expenditure towards fuel, lighting and housing.[37] It is also symptomatic of the extremely competitive conditions under which the growth in retail sales has taken place. The largest volume of sales is in food, but it is in this section that sales levels have been most stable, while expenditure on clothes and household accessories has increased dramatically.

Competition in retailing stems from three sources. The first is chain stores, comprising food supermarkets and specialist and general durable goods stores and owned by large chain stores, some of which have interests in wholesaling and manufacture. The second is small chains, largely made up of department stores. The third, single-outlet retailers, provides most mobility into and out of the industry. Because of the atomistic nature of the market-place, the customers' loyalty to all three types of company depends on price and quality. Collusion such as is possible in manufacturing does not exist in retailing, though co-operation in wholesale supply has become increasingly widespread among single-outlet retailers.

Up to 1971 there was an increased volume of sales in a declining number of stores, but with a small rate of increase in employment. During the 1970s the size of store units increased while both the number of employees and the value of sales levels declined. The causes were multifold. Large chain stores merged or were taken over, a move normally followed by rationalisation and renewal of sites and units. Self-service started in department stores and specialist chains. The number of locally owned and operated outlets fell sharply as a result of increased price competition from chains. Meanwhile, the respective shares of the market enjoyed by each mode of sales changed significantly, with the large chain stores attaining the bulk of the market.

During the 1980s, sales levels have increased in value, but gross margins remain small. Most major food chain stores reported profits of 2.5 per cent. A recent government inquiry reported a net return on retail sales of 1.3 per cent, with a loss of 3 per cent on clothing and footwear. Capital expenditure increased in the 1980s as a result of increases in site values and the reconstruction of sales outlets. This reflects a heightening competition for sites located in prime inner-city shopping centres or more especially for suburban hypermarkets (or superstores). In spite of slow growth, or perhaps because of it, the pace of re-organisation has been rapid. Increased concentration of control has not implied a slackening of competition. Indeed, competition, or rather contest, between the large chain stores has set the pace in both price and quality. The effect of this oligopolistic contest may be seen in the increased productivity during the 1970s and 1980s. It has also changed the nature of retail outlets quite dramatically; labour-intensive personal service stores have given place to serve-yourself displays manned largely by cashiers and shelf-fillers rather than by sales people.

Food retailing has changed in particular. One of the most important technological developments underlying this trend has been the introduction of new methods of food preservation, beginning with canning, then freezing and more recently with chemical preservatives. This ability to give a long shelf-life to products enables large quantities to be displayed in a way that provides the basis for the supermarket form of selling. Profitability still depends on a high volume of quick sales turnovers and carefully controlled buying. Large chain stores have centralised these functions in order to gain better discounts, and others rely heavily on sales of own-brand goods. Many of the owner-operated outlets belong to co-operative wholesale buying and packing groups or are run on a franchised basis. They do not succeed on the basis of price competition but on convenience of locality and long hours of opening. With demand for food static, several major chain stores have diversified into non-food goods for which margins are better. Some have become strong competitors against specialist food shops through widening their range of in-store departments.

The same trend, towards centralisation of ownership accompanied by diversification at the point of sale, may be observed across all sectors. Different styles of shops from own-label boutiques to discount warehouses are being promoted by the large chain stores in order to compete with new entrants. These latter are to be found in markets having rapid changes in fashion and based on new sources of supply. The production of designer clothes, for intance, draws from rapidly expanding supplies of home-workers in the garment industry, while furniture and household goods are imported from Eastern Europe and China where labour costs are lower than those of the United Kingdom.

Industrial relations and conditions of employment

At the present time most major chain stores have separate national agreements with the two major trade unions, the Union of Shop, Distributive and Allied Workers (USDAW) and the Transport and General Workers' Union (TGWU). Two industry-wide negotiating bodies were set up in 1974, one for food retailing, the other for non-food. They set minimum wage rates for five grades of salespersons, shelf-fillers and warehouse people stretching from general assistants (Grade Five) to supervisors or departmental manager (Grade One). Managers are not covered by the agreement.

Wider still in its coverage are the statutorily enforced minima of the Wages Councils, one for food, the other for non-food. These stemmed from the efforts of the Shop Assistants' Union and its political allies in 1906. Retailing was regarded then as the most significant example of exploited labour in "exploited trades". Only the Consumer Co-operative Movement recognised the union. In 1945 the Labour Government revised the legislation allowing the newly named USDAW to apply for a Wages Council, and large employers, realising the strength of competition from family shops, supported it.[38] Even so, several councils for each section of the industry fragmented the union's efforts until their amalgamation in 1974.

For many years USDAW was regarded as a house union in the Co-operative Movement. During the 1970s the reorganisation of the industry brought many private-sector employees into membership. This was accelerated when the TGWU extended its recruitment from delivery truck drivers and warehouse people to the sales floor. Eventually the TUC brought about a jurisdictional agreement between the two unions, but not before employees in major chain stores had made agreements with USDAW, some of them being post-entry closed shops or union shops with check-off arrangements. Where union shops do not exist, USDAW membership is only significant in menswear, consumer durables and other male-dominated sectors of employment. Elsewhere, national chain owners express satisfaction with an arrangement which allows a strongly paternalistic style of management in local stores while a negotiated national minimum rate of pay reduces wage competition in a highly labour-intensive industry.

The effect of agreements made in Wage Councils was to keep the statutory minimum rate (SMR) somewhat below the minimum rates determined across industry by collective bargaining up to 1969. By 1976 the SMR had fallen to 77 per cent of the minimum rates in the rest of industry. From that time onwards it has climbed, and for women was 10 per cent above the national average in 1982. A number of factors contributed to this trend besides the new national agreements. In the mid-1970s it was held back by incomes policy; removal of this constraint combined with equal pay legislation to bring about an increase in labour costs. Yet the relative position of shop assistants in terms of overall *earnings*, including bonuses and additional payments, is somewhat different. Women remain comparatively disadvantaged because of lack of bonus opportunities within these forms of employment (for example, grocery check-outs as against the sales positions in durable goods occupied by men), and because of their part-time status.

Wages Council orders cover only full-time workers: these are taken to be those working at least 36 hours a week. Normally, workers in chain stores work a 39-hour week distributed across six days and including at least one evening until 7 or 9 p.m. Employees working fewer than 28 hours per week are not covered by the provisions of the National Insurance Act and, therefore, the employer does not have to pay the 14 per cent of wages which constitute his statutory contribution. These two statutorily imposed minima form a structure for employment within the industry. Some smaller employers recruit full-time workers for less than 36 hours per week, but the trend across most of the industry is towards recruitment for less than 28 hours per week in all except the core occupations.

The number of part-time workers and the uses to which they are put vary. Grocery and Confectionery and Tobacco (CTN) appears to maintain the smallest core of full-time staff, department stores somewhat larger, and menswear, pharmacists and specialised chains the highest. In some stores, work is organised on a two- or three-shift system which enables the continuous deployment of part-time workers; in others, part-time workers constitute a "buffer" force for weekends, meal times and seasonal peaks.

An explanation for the differences may be found in the standardised nature of the goods sold or the need for specialised after-sales service and knowledge of the product on the part of the salesperson. For example, check-out operators in supermarkets need little product knowledge (in theory at least), while "white goods" sales people need to know something of the electromechanical functioning of refrigerators and ovens (again in theory).

In addition to part-time workers there are firms of concessionaires occupying space to sell specialised products in department stores and largely employed by producers. In supermarkets there is a similar group of self-employed merchandisers who are hired by high-profit product manufacturers like confectionery and cosmetics to travel from store to store replenishing shelves. Both forms of employment are increasing as store owners seek to reduce their overhead labour costs.

The major constraint on hours of work is the statutory regulations governing hours of opening. These were originally passed as an indirect means of improving employee conditions. However, they are now supported by small traders for whom they operate in a way that offers them an advantage over chain stores, for while the regulations can be

111

easily enforced in shopping centres, they are generally not rigorously imposed on neighbourhood shops.

Electronic point of sale (EPOS)

There are basically three levels of sophistication in computerised sales-based systems available to retailers:

- electronic cash registers (ECRs) which perform almost exactly the same work as the electromechanical units they are due to replace;
- at a more sophisticated level, the "stand-alone data-capture units" which perform all the normal functions of a cash register but also record information about sales on an internal magnetic tape cassette which can be removed and processed at appropriate time intervals;
- the most sophisticated level of point-of-sale units, those which are fully linked to a computer-controlled system and which may incorporate laser scanning. (These will normally be referred to as EPOS – electronic point-of-sale equipment unless otherwise indicated.)

The focus of this section is upon the third, most sophisticated level, where point-of-sale terminals potentially form the "front end" of totally integrated computer-based retailing systems. It is a system designed to control large turnovers of diversified stock and, in the first installations, it provided extensions to an already centralised data bank of the kind already described in banking.

EPOS were first introduced in the United States in the early 1970s as a means of integrating buying operations with sales, in a manner that reduced the need for stock holding and provided a machine-imposed discipline on the labour process. It was made possible by the development of integrated electronic circuitry and its inclusion in minicomputers which could be linked to a central mainframe computer. By magnetic wanding, laser scanning or keying-in of coded details, itemised commodities could be monitored and controlled centrally across any number of sales outlets, however geographically remote. It also provided the possibility of automatic adjustment of subsystem requirements, particularly stock replenishment or reordering from manufacturers, without human intervention.

Of more immediate relevance to pioneering users of EPOS was the production of the operational information and analysis of day-to-day (minute-to-minute) operations which enabled better resource allocation to be carried out by local management and better central monitoring of sales and stocks. The first users in Europe were the Modena Co-operative

Society in Italy, and a department store (Breuniger) in Stuttgart – in both cases, single-store installations were made in 1973. In the United Kingdom the first users were Goldbergs in Glasgow, and the John Lewis chain and the Lewis chain of department stores (separate enterprises), both of which introduced EPOS on an incremental, store-by-store basis, using the first installation as a pilot for the second, and so on. By the mid-1970s, 20 stores had installed EPOS in Western Europe; over 20,000 existed in the United States. In 1985, there were only 167 stores using EPOS in the United Kingdom, although the largest chains are now committed to install the system in all new stores.

The slow take-up of EPOS can be explained by the high cost of installation which in the early period doubled the investment for a new superstore. In the last three years these costs have fallen by 30 per cent and are continuing to fall rapidly. One reason for the reduction in cost is the increased reliability of the system, which diminishes the need for the duplication of cabled circuits and dual storage capacity. The main cause of delayed investment was the time taken by British and other European manufacturers to agree on the type of bar coding to be used in labelling goods in order to record their name and source by passing them over a laser beam. Even after agreement on a European Article Numbering System, it has taken five years for most manufacturers to adopt it. Early users of EPOS were forced to mark their own goods upon receipt from the manufacturer. This is still the case for many consumer durables such as garments, but in packaged and canned foods nearly all manufacturers throughout the world code their goods at source.

EPOS is currently designed around two formats, illustrated in figure 3 below. In the format used in supermarkets, goods are passed over a laser beam covered with glass and onto a loading tray in the manner of normal check-outs. In durable goods shops and department stores, the cashier passes a hand-held wand across the magnetic code printed on a ticket or label attached to the purchased article. The code activates a signal to the itemised price schedule contained in the memory of the EPOS till or in the store controller computer, depending on the system, and the price flashes on a screen displayed to the customer. The keyboard is made up of numbers pressed to indicate the codes of articles which do not have a bar or magnetic code printed on them, and other keys which automatically register the codes of the most popular unlabelled items, such as bread.

Price item schedules are normally fed into the local store computer from a central (head office or regional centre) computer by on-line connection once a week, or whenever changes occur. They are printed in price manual format by the central computer. Updates to the manual are dispatched by road delivery service to coincide with changes in the

Figure 3 EPOS formats

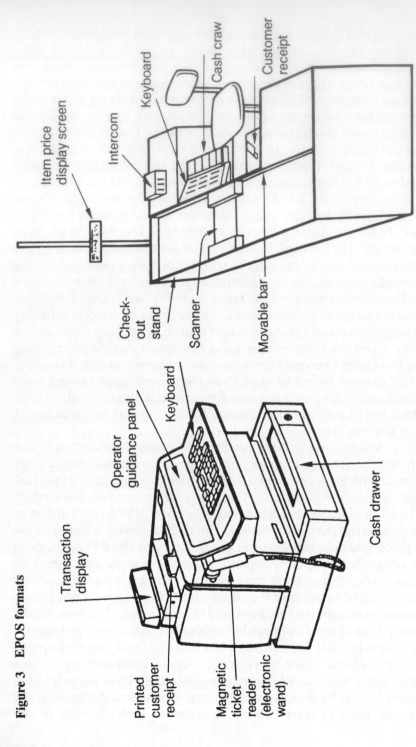

Item price display screen

Intercom

Keyboard

Cash craw

Customer receipt

Scanner

Check-out stand

Movable bar

Electronic scanner at supermarket check-out

Transaction display

Operator guidance panel

Keyboard

Printed customer receipt

Magnetic ticket reader (electronic wand)

Cash drawer

Point-of-sale terminal in department store

computer data base. The manuals should be available to cashiers or check-out operators for use in handling customer queries or other problems.

In a complementary process the item prices are printed on shelf-edge labels and dispatched to local stores. One of the major cost savings in the utilisation of EPOS in supermarkets is that on price-labelling each item. Price labelling was formerly done by hand, each price revision involved removing or covering up existing prices with a stick-on label. This labour-intensive exercise is replaced by affixing a single plastic label in front of a stack of unmarked goods, a modification which required a change in the British law on consumer protection. The statute still requires all goods to be stacked separately behind the correct sale price so that great care has to be taken to change all shelf labels at the time that EPOS check-out terminals are reprogrammed. This saving is not usually available to stores selling durable goods, which normally have prices visually labelled on each individual item.

The records of transactions are stored in a master computer in the store (often one of the EPOS terminals in master/slave relationship with the others) and can be cabled back to the central computer at the end of each day or dispatched on magnetic tape at longer intervals, depending on whether a real-time or batch-processing system is being used at the head office or regional office. These are utilised in a number of ways. The most basic use is in the keeping and auditing of accounts: sales can be compared on an itemised basis with invoices received from suppliers and with dispatch notes from the regional depots. These invoices and notes may be the only record of the receipt of goods by the local stores or, in a fully integrated information system, they may simply verify computer entries made by the warehouse or depot dispatcher and by the receiver (goods-in clerk) in the stockroom of the local store.

The more strategic use of EPOS-generated data is in the design of sales and purchasing policies. The first allows goods to be stacked in a variety of positions within the shop until the variation in sales data indicates an optimal distribution. The same data can be used to assess sales promotion and allocation of products throughout the country. Of more importance to labour costs, the system renders exact detail on the flow of transactions over any measured period.

The system can show when more or less labour is required, and the time taken for each transaction can be measured together with its content. On the basis of the flow data the staffing system (including the arrangement of shifts) can be controlled with great accuracy. With the transaction data much greater discipline can be asserted in the management of local workers by the head office.

Perhaps the greatest promise from EPOS was the prospect of an integrated retailing system. The key to this lies in automatic reordering of goods on the basis of current sales and current stocks (purchase order management). This system operates in the United States to ensure the automatic refurbishing of stockrooms from company depots, and often to activate fresh deliveries from producers or wholesalers without the intervention of a (human) company buyer. It does not operate in Europe, where the sales information is used solely as a guide by head office buyers in their purchase of labelled goods and by local managers in obtaining fresh foods from local suppliers.

A number of personal service chain stores have resisted EPOS because they prefer to rely on the qualitative information obtained from salespersons on customer preferences, particularly on what the customer would have preferred to purchase but could not because it was not on the shelves. It remains true that the detailed sales data obtained from EPOS and the analysis to which it can be submitted has radically changed the intuitive nature of the buying function. This is more true of the bulk purchasing of foods for supermarkets than for the buying of fashion garments and household goods, where customer tastes can be volatile. Even here, the use of day-to-day records of sales can enable the buyer who has placed preliminary orders with a seller employing 200 home-based workshops, to determine within days rather than weeks which half-dozen will remain in work. A typical sequential work flow is set out in figure 4.

Other electronic data processing developments

Single outlets or small chains are beginning to invest in second-level data-capture machines. The tapes from these can be processed by computer agencies who collect them on a daily or weekly basis and return print-outs of sales analyses on an agreed basis. The use of microcomputers is much more widespread to produce spreadsheets on the basis of data transferred from ordinary till rolls. Both uses help small retailers to be more efficient, but the most significant long-term effects come through the uses to which EDP is being put by large chain stores.

These range from apparently small developments, such as portable data capture units (PDCs) to home shopping via telematics. PDCs are currently used in conjunction with EPOS systems or as substitutes for them to record stocks and flows of goods from the retailer's or supplier's depot to the shop or store warehouse and while on the sales shelves. They can equally well be used to record and transmit flows of cash. The operator

Figure 4   Sequential work flow in integrated retailing system

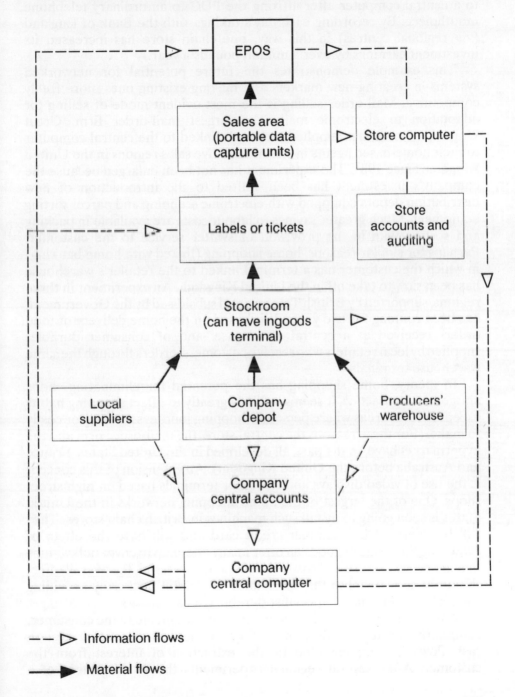

Legend:

--- ▷ Information flows

�merchantarrow Material flows

keys in data on a hand-held machine which is recorded and played back to a central computer after affixing the PDC to an ordinary telephone mouthpiece. By recording each day's takings with the Bank of England (via regional centres) in this way, one chain store has increased its investment earnings by over a million pounds a year.

This example demonstrates the future potential for networked systems in creating new markets and making existing ones more freely competitive. Mail-order selling is the most evident mode of selling for adaptation to electronic mail. The largest mail-order firm, Great Universal Stores, has supplied terminals linked to the central computer to their home-based agents in one of their five sales regions in the United Kingdom since 1981. The experiment has not been enlarged because the company's investment has been shifted to the introduction of new distribution depots equipped with electronic scanning and parcel sorting equipment. Much greater savings in labour costs are available in packing and sorting than in the provision of swifter service to the customer. Perhaps for similar reasons, home shopping (linked with home banking) in which the customer has a terminal linked to the retailer's warehouse has been slow to take off in the United Kingdom. An experiment in three regions, supported by British Telecom and subsidised by the Government, has been running for two years. It is based on the home delivery of food orders received at a central warehouse, and of consumer durables supplied by local retailers who receive customers' orders through the same warehouse terminals.

In theory, home shopping has the potential for eliminating shops altogether. In practice, it seems unlikely greatly to affect shopping habits except in rural areas where personal shopping journeys are long or costly to make. (For these reasons the central store, the mail-order firm and the hypermarket have, in the past, all developed in the United States, France and Australia before the United Kingdom). An extension of this concept is the use of video displays and customer terminals based on high street shops. One of the largest of the home shopping networks in the United States is soon going to install such machines in British chain stores. They will be operated by customer credit card and will have the effect of extending the range of goods on offer in any one shop to cover bulky items that are costly to store and costly to deliver. If successful, the overall effect should be to rationalise the distribution chain still further by providing cut-cost competition for specialist durable goods retailers.

As cost cutting comes close to the margin acceptable to the consumer, competitive strategy moves into the financial field. The use of interest on cash flows is complemented by the extraction of interest from the customer. After several regional experiments the establishment of a national Eftpos (Electronic Funds Transfer at the Point of Sale) has been announced in which a consortium of chain stores has agreed on a scheme with the clearing banks and major building societies which will allow shoppers at stores using EPOS systems to pay by directly debiting their bank accounts or credit card account. IBM is to design and implement the first phase of the system in collaboration with British Telecom. A number of major chains including Marks & Spencer have already initiated their own credit card system in collaboration with banks or finance houses. Estimates of the scheme's impact are still modest at 12 per cent of sales by 1996.

Case studies of two department stores

Two chains of department stores were studied, one large (12 branches) and the other small (two branches). In 1980 the large chain employed 5,000 people, having reduced its staff from 20,000 in 1970. Turnover increased from 75 million to 100 million over the same period. The increase in productivity was achieved through a switch to self-service and through the replacement of full-time by part-time employees. This was accomplished through natural wastage. By the end of the decade a conflict between the store sales managers and the head office buyers in the company had been exacerbated by the lack of qualitative information derived from their reduced staff. The rather late purchase of a central computer in 1977 led to a first integration of the sales and buying functions. Then, takeover by a group of shoe manufacturers led to a further centralisation of data analysis at regional computer centres using daily returns from cash registers delivered by road to the centres. The need to replace old cash registers precipitated a decision to invest in EPOS. It was not seen as a means to rationalise labour costs, but rather as a means to cope with a sales information problem that had been exacerbated by previous rationalisation. Nevertheless, in the cases we observed, 200 old cash registers were replaced by 65 EPOS terminals on each site and evident staff reductions had resulted.

Stores were converted one at a time, and experience gained in one was transferred to another. Staff were informed that "new tills" were to be installed six months before they were fitted, and national trade union (USDAW) representatives were invited to see the original sites. Training for salespersons was undertaken by 12 junior managers recruited for the purpose and themselves trained by the manufacturer, IBM. Some terminals were set up in a training area in each store, and all sales staff were given a minimum of 15 hours of training. Shop stewards were briefed only after sufficient staff had been trained for their members' commitment to the new system to be ensured. Accounts clerks were trained for six weeks, including a one-week IBM residential course.

In a departmental breakdown of experience, EPOS could be seen to have brought about potential changes in career and task conditions, many of which had still to be implemented. In a typical department, staff had reduced from 24, 16 of whom were full-time, to 17, all but two (the managers) of whom were part-time. At the time of our initial study, the salesperson and cashier roles remained as a single occupation. The company experimented with a special cashier role for two years in their Liverpool store before propagating this new division of labour throughout the group. The change was generally welcomed by staff, who had found that the EPOS terminals took longer to operate than the previous cash registers and were, therefore, creating bottle-necks at peak periods. (It seems likely to the authors that customer queues were created by the reduction in the number of cash points rather than the operational speed of EPOS.) Nevertheless, the change brought about a dual career for shop-floor workers which leads to different end positions as chief cashier for the whole store, or as departmental manager, a position normally occupied by a man. Cashiers were now managed by a chief cashier whose position in some respects was senior to that of the departmental managers to whom cashiers reported on a day-to-day basis. This was not the only function to be removed from the departmental manager. Functional control over both stock and customer credit was moving upwards in the hierarchy and the head office systems department saw display and lay-out as being progressively directed by their analysis of sales data.

The accounts and audit department has greatly extended its control over store operations and over communications with the head office. This has been achieved through its usurpation of both the price-ticketing department (pre-sales) and the store's computer access to the regional office. The major staffing reductions occurred in auditing (20 down to five) which also became the key link in the computer system. Previously, the staff had engaged in the collection and collation of paper rolls from each of the 200 tills spread across some 50 departments on a daily basis. Now departmental managers collect till rolls from those cash registers still in use (in fresh foods and concessionaires). These are still entered into the store computer, along with the automatically stored data from the EPOS terminals. Vouchers for cash received from cashiers are checked against EPOS and cash register receipts; separate accounts are made up for the self-employed concessionaires who also occupy space within the store. Two people are employed full-time in checking deficits and surpluses in receipts. In this way an overall master record is kept in the store as well as at the regional level. The most important change to have occurred was in the work of two senior cashiers who had become responsible for entering the information in the computer onto the regional machine each evening (when the telephone link is cheapest). This consisted of the day's EPOS records, together with the integrated (cash register and EPOS) data of the previous day. They were women in their late 50s, one a widow, the other single, who enjoyed the long hours at the overtime rate. One had been given formal promotion from cashier to senior cashier; the other had not, but was paid at the higher rate because it was company policy to have no more than one senior cashier.

The other major departmental change had come through the establishment of a central price labelling or pre-retail department, which had taken over the task of ticketing goods from sales staff in each separate department. This change had been initiated before the introduction of computers in 1976, but price-item schedules are now obtained from the regional computer via a VDU in the pre-retail department. The magnetic tags are manually printed, according to instructions received, and attached to the goods by hand. In this way the salesperson cannot alter prices, and the departmental manager cannot engage in special promotions.

Staff reaction to the changes brought about by EPOS were largely subsumed by more basic fears of redundancy among long-serving employees, of a takeover that occurred in 1980 and of general moves toward rationalisation and centralisation. These fears were not shared by recently recruited staff, mainly school-leavers glad of any kind of employment. Trade union consultation was minimal. It was not until after the change had taken place that USDAW made serious attempts to acquaint their representatives of the nature and implications of EPOS. Even then it seemed to the authors that trade union officers saw little basis for a strategic response. Within management, the data-processing department had become the major influence in the ongoing re-organisation of the company, supervised by the financial directorate. Departmental managers within each store lost the most autonomy and influence. Store managers themselves were under some degree of threat. There appeared to be a widespread inability to use the comprehensive analyses produced by the head office to guide them. They, like the sales managers, preferred to rely on their "feel" for the market.

Within the small chain the same process could be observed on a much reduced scale. Few staff reductions among the 36 sales employees had yet occurred over the four-year span of operations, but older staff were to be phased out on retirement over the next two years. The system had been introduced by a company secretary (accountant) specifically recruited by the family owners of the business to install a computerised system. In fact, the system brought together data on stocks and flows of materials across a variety of small businesses owned by the family, including timber yards and a small deep-sea wharf and warehouse.

As in the large chain, some salespeople (one in this case, possibly as many as 100 in the larger store) left because they believed themselves too old to grasp "the new system". It is important to note that it was not the operation of the terminal itself that was difficult, but the failure to understand, and the consequent fear of, the conceptual system of which the terminal was part. A more widespread discontent among salespersons derived from the elimination of written invoices and handwritten ledgers. These had previously been taken to a specialised cashier. Now the salespersons operated the tills as well as assisted customers with their purchases, so that they could no longer concentrate on the latter role. This is a change of role that was counter to that in the larger company. It indicated, as do differences between shops within the same chain, that the response to the same technology can be very different – indeed, a directly opposite one.

Case study of a supermarket

This supermarket is prototypical of the macro changes in the industry. It was formed by a processor of frozen foods from an amalgamation of small chains and independent groceries totalling 113 outlets, only seven of which might be categorised as a supermarket in terms of area (over 25,000 square feet). In 1983 it was sold by the original founders to a food group which since that time has taken over three other chains in order to create a chain of 740 outlets, the fifth largest chain in the country.

The EPOS system was installed in three stores between 1979 and 1980, and ten more installations were to have been made in the new stores. In fact the stores were not built, and on being taken over by the larger group, one of the three EPOS stores was sold, while three more were acquired with other groups. The five stores were all re-equipped with new Japanese equipment which was believed to be more reliable and which could be interfaced with the variety of central mainframe computers around which the system was to be organised.

The new owners modified the basis of the system, moving from an on-line to a batch system of processing in which price-item schedules are received by cable at the store but sales data are collected on tape by delivery van each day and print-outs received back from the head office by local managers once a week. Local store managers are encouraged to do their own sales analysis on personal computers. All but the existing five stores are being equipped with electronic cash registers (of the first grade of sophistication). These produce sales results on magnetic tape. The sales tapes can be inserted into personal computers and can be recorded by local managers before being collected for later analysis at the head office. The analysis produced in this way is not as detailed as that created by the EPOS form of recording, so the five stores are to be retained as experimental controls in the reorganisation of sales and introduction of new products.

Clearly, this represents a step backwards in technology, but one which has gone along with the introduction of a number of intermediate forms of information technology. For example, mobile data-capture units are used to make daily checks of stock on shelves and in the stockroom. This information is conveyed to the regional depots by telephone each day, and forms the basis of the stock replenishment system, together with orders received from departmental managers. The company is also experimenting with buying commodities via a telex (cabled) system or requesting daily tenders from suppliers of vegetables and fruit within easy access for delivery. The regional buyer can select the most favoured bid in a televisual auction.

The changed pattern of jobs in EPOS stores resembles that in the department store, except that it revolves around the already specialised function of cashier or check-out operator. Other shop-floor jobs that were changed were those of shelf-filling and labelling (the lowest grades of pay) in a way that has already been described. A pre-retail price coding group of workers was created during the first eighteen months of operations, consisting of seven part-time employees who stood in line around a conveyor belt unpacking cartons of packaged foods and printing a bar code on each item with hand-held guns. A laser scanner at the end of the line was used to check each item before it was stacked in a pannier for shelf-filling. These people were redeployed as more and more goods were pre-coded by manufacturers.

The major changes in tasks were, as in department stores, in the "back office". The records from each terminal are checked with cash drawers from the check-outs at the end of each shift, by means of a VDU in the cashier's office rather than against till rolls. Only four people (two part-time) are employed to keep accounts for the store, which has 14 check-out terminals and an annual sales turnover of 10 million. No change has been made in the staff, but a head office systems manager based in the store during the first two years of operations has been made redundant. Consequently, communication with the head office computer installation, including the receipt of price labels, is through the computer office. However, a new appointment of front-end manager has been made to check price-item schedules, to supervise the check-out operators (including training new staff) and to supervise shelf-edge labelling. The occupant of the role is the wife of the redundant systems manager who was first engaged to train check-out operators within the company as a whole. She is now the most expert person in the store in the systems operation.

The reaction of the check-out operators to the introduction of EPOS was mixed. It became focused on the change in evening shifts that resulted from head office analysis of sales results. There was a spontaneous collective protest, but when their shop steward, who was departmental manager, refused to take up their grievance, the objection was not pursued. Subsequently, the national union representatives have visited the store with management from other stores considering EPOS, with evident approval.

As in the department store, opinion was divided between long-service workers and new recruits. By and large, such is the rationalisation of staff that few people remain for a long time on EPOS terminals or use VDUs for long periods except on weekends and other peak periods. Everyone, including the departmental managers, perform many tasks and are used according to their ability rather than according to their grade of pay. It is this move towards greater polyvalent use of labour that predominates, rather than the impact of EPOS at store level. Other developments such as automated meat cutting and packing have deprived tradesmen like butchers of the ability to use their skills. These developments can be related to the needs of standardisation and pre-pricing, but are proceeding separately.

Summary of the case studies

The effects of EPOS have been to alleviate some of the stresses caused by the existing rationalisation of staff and to increase flexibility in the use of employees across several tasks on the shop floor. Staff reactions have been tempered by their position in a rapidly deteriorating labour market. In general, many of the complaints appeared to relate to increased workloads brought about through the rationalisation in staff numbers and equipment rather than by the equipment itself. The major changes that have not been described or observed by the authors in detail are those taking place in headquarters staff. This is difficult to analyse because company takeovers and mergers have led to a wholesale dismissal of staff or to their dispersal over sites in one or another of the acquired companies.

Clearly, the number of data-processing staff grouped around main-frame computers has tended to grow, despite temporary setbacks and reorganisation designed to reduce their influence. Their systematic approach proves challenging to existing managers, particularly management at the point of service. Sales managers may lose their information-gathering and information-processing function by the new ability at the centre of the company to obtain and analyse data over a much wider area of the company's operations, and with the statistically modelled expertise contained in the information technology.

The jobs of large numbers of (mostly female) clerks employed in head office audit departments to match invoices to receipts are clearly at risk. At present, these paper transactions are checked with the central computer's records of sales and stocks. None of the pioneer users of EPOS has yet adopted a fully integrated system in which dispatches and receipts are solely recorded on computer terminals at warehouses, depots and stockrooms and matched with sales records from point-of-sale machines. For this to occur, greater trust would be required between suppliers and purchasers in the distribution chain, but the labour cost saving would be considerable.

The impact of microelectronics in hospitals, banking and retailing

Our observations tend to support a pessimistic view of the effects of information technology on the occupational structure and working conditions of employees in these three sectors. This impression is by no means universal, uni-directional or attributable to the use of new technology per se. Throughout all three sections of the service economy, we have observed conditions of increased contest for resources and rationalisation of expenditure, accompanied by a growing attempt to assert central standards of control and discipline at the point of service. We might indeed be witnessing a trend towards the industrialisation of service work in which new technology is playing no more than an enabling role. It might well be asked if the changes brought about by employers' reactions to economic crises are to have a permanent effect.

In some cases, it is difficult to discern a trend in the design of new jobs because line managers as yet retain some autonomy to experiment in their use of labour and, in some cases, the company or organisation has deliberately set out to encourage a diversity of approaches to new technology. Often the influence of the occupations around which the internal hierarchy revolves has been powerful enough to resist the mounting pressures towards central control. The hypothesis with which we began our project has proved a fruitful one. In the National Health Service the standing of doctors made them the prime movers of technological innovation from the introduction of computers in the 1960s. It has, in fact, taken the direct intervention of the government to impose a new managerial structure on the allocation of resources and budgeting of health care finances in a way that has shifted control over both new investment and over the focus of this investment to the centre of the NHS. Less dramatic, but nevertheless as inexorable, has been the movement away from the autonomy previously enjoyed by the bank manager and the retail store manager to the centre of firms in these sectors.

Throughout this power struggle, information technology has provided organisational designers with options for greater or less involvement of line operators and consumers. *There has never been a technologically determined answer to the question of who should control the computer terminal.* By and large those groups and individuals that have knowledge and skills related to the existing system, and who have been willing to adopt the language of the computer, have found new influence. Often, however, because they are stigmatised by gender, this technical influence is not recognised in their present level of rewards or, more importantly, in their promotion opportunities. The newly emerging young computer-trained managers are quite consciously selected from among male aspirants rather than female. We are forced to the conclusion that many of the temporary gains in employment conditions achieved by a minority of women will not be permanent ones.

The period of negotiated learning during which male line managers come to terms with the new concepts and new skills required to communicate through a terminal will allow some upgrading of "women's jobs". We see little likelihood of unions being able – or anxious – to secure monopolies over these skills in the way that male craft unions have in previous eras. In the long run it seems likely that the shift to a centrally determined organisational rationale focused on cost-effectiveness will lead to an increasing polarisation of jobs and of conditions of work in the service sector.

It seems equally likely that the contest for part-time or casual work may become greater across the economy as a whole, particularly if the present economic decline continues. That being so, a new factor in the status of marginalised jobs may be the growing recruitment of males to such jobs. This would also be a factor in determining the future reconstruction of skills at the point of service delivery, given their greater propensity to join and be active in trade unions and professional associations.

Notes

* In this report, the section on banking was contributed by John Child, that on retailing by Ray Loveridge, and that on health care by Janet Harvey. Ray Loveridge undertook overall editing.

1 See, for example, D. Bell: *Work and its discontents* (New York, League for Industrial Democracy, 1970); and R. Bolt: "Man-machine partnership", in J.G. Burke (ed.): *The new technology and human values* (Belmont, California, Wadsworth, 1966).

2 C. Hakim: "Occupational segregation: A comparative study of the degree and pattern of the differentiation between men and women's work in Britain, the United States and other countries", in *Department of Employment Research Paper No. 9* (London, Nov. 1979).

3 K. Marx: *Capital*, Vol. I (trans. B. Fowkes) (Harmondsworth, Penguin, 1867, 1976 ed.).

4 H. Braverman: *Labor and monopoly capital* (New York, Monthly Review Press, 1974).

5 Bell, op. cit.; Bolt, op. cit.

6 An aggregate investment figure for new technology is not available, since such spending is devolved to the regions and comes from their general budgetary allocation.

7 In terms of gross domestic product (GDP), this represents a percentage rise of expenditure on health care from 3.9 per cent in 1949 to 6.1 per cent in 1980.

8 I. Illich: *Medical nemesis: The expropriation of health* (Calder and Boyars, 1975) (revised in 1976 as *Limits to medicine*).

9 T. Rathwell, A.F. Long and A.D. Clayden: "Computing development and education for management in the NHS", in *Hospital and Health Service Review*, Vol. 79, No. 6, Nov. 1983, pp. 266-267.

10 R. Griffiths: *NHS management enquiry document* (6 Oct. 1983).

11 DHSS: *Reports 1-6, Steering Group of Health Service Information*, Chair: Mrs. E. Korner (1982).

12 Cf. W. Rogers, B. Ryack and G. Moeller: "Computer-aided medical diagnosis: Literature review", in *International Journal of Biomedical Computing*, 10, 1979, pp. 267-287.

13 K. Clarke Hansard: *MLSOs – England as at 30 September 1983 – Gender and hierarchical breakdown*, Written Answers, 3 June 1985, p. 106.

14 H. Homans: *Equal opportunities in the NHS: A case study of laboratory staff* (forthcoming HMSO publication).

15 Sir T. Bevan: "Address to the 7th Annual Conference of the Clearing Bank Union", reported in *Interest*, Dec. 1984: 2.

16 Department of Employment: *Gazette*, Historical Supplement No. 1, Aug. 1984.

17 J. Child and N. Tarbuck: "The introduction of new technologies: Managerial initiative and union response in British banks", in *Industrial Relations Journal* (Nottingham), Vol. 16, No. 3, Autumn 1985, pp. 19-33.

18 A. Rajan: *New technology and employment in insurance, banking and building societies: Recent experience and future impact* (Aldershot, Gower, 1984).

19 Banking Information Services: *The banks and information technology* (1982).

20 J. Marti and A. Zeillinger: *Micros and money: New technology in banking and shopping* (London, Policy Studies Institute, 1982).

21 "Technological Change", in *Banking World* (Oxford, Pergamon Press), Nov. 1984, pp. 43-51.

22 J. Child and M. Tarbuck, op. cit.

23 B. Clement: "Bank union fears tills will mean redundancy", in *The Times*, 24 Sept. 1984, p. 2; and B. Riley: "Automation is the key to six-day opening at Nat West", in *Financial Times*, 14 Sept. 1984, p. 8.

24 Cf. P. Willman and R. Cowan: "New technology in banking: The impact of autotellers on staff numbers", in M. Warner (ed.): *Microprocessors, manpower and society* (Aldershot, Gower, 1984).

25 Cf. T. Nicholas: "Effects on retail banking", in *The banks and technology in the 1980s* (London, Institute of Bankers, 1982).

26 A. Rajan, op. cit.

27 P. Willman and R. Cowan, op. cit.

28 B. Groom: "Technology is cutting full-time bank staff", in *Financial Times*, 15 Apr. 1985, p. 8.

29 See, for example, A. Egan: "Women in banking: A study in inequality", in *Industrial Relations Journal* (Nottingham), Vol. 13, No. 3, 1982, Issue 13, pp. 20-31.

30 Cf. S. Smith: *Work organisation, gender and technical change in banking: The social limits of scientific management*. Paper given to the 3rd Annual Aston-UMIST Conference on the Labour Process (Manchester, Apr. 1985).

31 ibid.

32 R. Farley, as reported in *Banking World* (Oxford, Pergamon Press), May 1984, p. 18.

33 J. Child: "New technology and the 'service class'", in S. Allen *et al.* (eds): *The changing experience of work* (London, Macmillan, 1986).

34 See J. Child and M. Tarbuck, op. cit.

35 B. Hedberg and M. Mehlmann: *Tomorrow's bank: Seven pictures of Swedish banks in 1990* (Stockholm, Swedish Centre for Working Life, 1982).

36 J. Child, R. Loveridge, J. Harvey and A. Spencer: "Microelectronics and the quality of employment in services", in P. Marstrand (ed.): *New technology and the future of work and skills* (London, Frances Pinter, 1984).

37 C. Craig and F. Wilkinson: *Pay and employment in four retail trades (Research paper No. 51)* (London, Department of Employment, 1985).

38 F.J. Bayliss: *British Wages Councils* (Oxford, Blackwells, 1962).

5 Advanced technology in offices and commerce in Japan

M. MINE

Common trends and background

Characteristics of office work in Japan

Today various kinds of new technology are being used in industry, but only the combined computer and telecommunication technology has a visible influence on Japanese society.

Offices in Japan differ from those in Western countries socially and organisationally. These differences affect the way new technology is applied. First of all, there is the Japanese writing system. It is a combination of ideograms (Chinese characters) and phonograms (the Japanese syllabary). Japanese typewriters, which only trained typists can use, have not always been used widely in daily business. Similarly, because it took time to develop word processors which can deal with the thousands of Japanese symbols, the facsimile network, which transmits visual information, is much more widespread than electronic mail, which connects word processors and keyboard-based terminals. Typewriters have disappeared from most offices in recent years and there has been a sharp increase in the use of word processors, as indicated in figure 1.

A second major difference is the group-oriented organisation of work in offices. *Ringi*, a group-centred decision-making process, is widely practised. Except for a few top-level managers, white-collar workers usually work in a common office space with their colleagues. The tasks of a section or a subsection are often distributed among its members fluidly. Occupational demarcations are obscure. The group-oriented nature of work organisation in Japan partly explains the infrequent friction during the process of technological change.

Office work in Japan is similar to that of other countries in that there are many simple jobs which can be replaced by computerised systems or by office automation machines (OA machines). Some of these systems

129

Figure 1   Sales of Japanese word processors

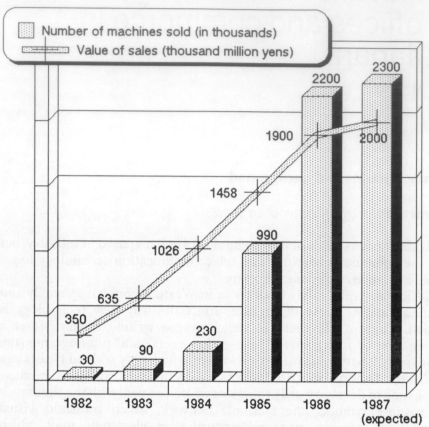

Source: *Nikkei OA Neuken* (Nikkei's OA Yearbook), 1988.

and machines can be used to support research or decision-making by employees in high positions, but many surveys indicate that the main purpose of the innovations is to raise the efficiency of office work.

Industrial relations and employment

Trade unions in Japan are mostly organised within companies. Under company-wide unionism, union members are likely to identify themselves with the enterprise which employs them. Trade unions in private industry generally support or at least do not oppose the introduction of new

130

technology. This is probably because company unions are aware of their competitive positions. In the public sector, where economic forces work indirectly, the attitudes of unions are not always co-operative towards management.

Most unions have been trying to promote joint consultations prior to any technological change. The major issues of interest to trade unions are employment security, transfers, training, and safety and health. According to a 1983 survey by the Ministry of Labour on the effects of office automation, 36 per cent of private unions were consulted by management prior to implementation of changes. These consultations rarely lead to written agreements between the parties.

Cases where office workers were discharged because of the introduction of new technology are almost unknown. One of the major reasons why trade unions accept technological change is employment security. Another reason is the practice by which workers who are transferred to other positions or whose assignments are changed by new technology are guaranteed their former wages. In Japan, wages are not strictly related to jobs; rather, they are seniority-oriented. The systems of wage payment in individual firms have scarcely changed, according to the above survey by the Ministry of Labour and other studies.

Under the lifetime employment plan of regular employees, adjustments of the workforce due to technological change are made mostly by controlling recruitment and by training and transferring employees. The Ministry of Labour survey reported minor employment changes due to the introduction of OA machines. The number of newly employed workers increased in the categories of new male college graduates and experienced workers, and decreased in the category of female high school graduates. The survey by the Ministry of Labour also reported that almost all companies provided some training for their workers in office automation, although three-quarters of the trained workers felt that their training was inadequate.

Social and economic changes

Japan is now experiencing radical social changes. In addition to technological innovations, the population is rapidly ageing and the participation of women in the labour force is increasing. The majority of women workers have unskilled jobs and can be replaced by microelectronic technology. New job opportunities are developing in the tertiary industries, but a substantial number of women workers will remain employed as unskilled part-time workers. Some may specialise in simple, repetitive jobs. These circumstances may lead to difficulties in raising the employment status or job satisfaction of women workers. The economy is also undergoing structural changes. The growth rate of the economy of Japan has tapered off since the oil crisis. Employers are much more concerned about the efficiency of their organisation than before, and public finance deficits have brought about administrative and financial reform plans directed toward low-cost government. The application of new technology has been promoted to keep labour costs at a minimum. This is reflected in such practices as contracting out keypunchers' jobs and operating computers around the clock. It may be difficult under the current economic conditions to balance the demands of employers for increased productivity through technology with the demands of employees for shorter working hours.

Consumers are more selective today and suppliers are obliged to respond instantly to their changing demands. The companies producing consumer goods have to manufacture many items with different specifications in small volume. A computerised communication network is becoming an indispensable means of doing business.

Technological developments

As semi-conductor technology developed, the potential of computers has expanded while price relative to performance has decreased. Telecommunication technology is shifting from analog to digital, greatly increasing the amount of information which can be sent over cables. Large firms with ample financial resources have led the way in introducing new equipment. Medium and small-sized firms have then followed their example in installing and using the new technology.

In Japan, a few large firms started using general-purpose computers for batch processing of office work in the late 1950s and early 1960s. Since then numerous repetitive office tasks, such as calculating wages, have been processed by computers at head offices. Since the 1970s an increasing number of large and medium-sized firms have established on-line systems, which consist of host computers linked to terminals.

Clerical tasks related to core business activities, namely sales, production, stocking and purchasing of commodities, are usually processed by on-line systems in large and medium-sized firms. Computers are also used in personnel management and accounting and are indispensable tools in research and design.

On-line systems provide advantages suited to business practices. Individual data-processing systems, which originally aimed at improving the efficiency of particular jobs, can be linked to create a total computerised network covering all relevant data of the firm. Several computers in each division can also be connected to form a network. Recently, some firms have connected their computers with those of other firms, subsidiary companies, customers, suppliers, banks, warehouses, and so on.

The current systematisation is accompanied in many cases by decentralised data processing. So-called "intelligent" terminals can process data locally and communicate the necessary information to host computers. A few industries have also introduced on-line systems in which terminals are specialised. Cash dispensers in banking and point-of-sale (POS) systems in the retail trade are well known.

An increasing number of word processors, personal computers, facsimile machines, and other machines equipped with microprocessors have been introduced in the past several years to deal with such jobs as the processing of irregular or infrequent standardised text, personal correspondence or data expressed in graphs. The majority of these machines are used on a stand-alone basis. However, networks of OA machines controlled by specialised computers or networks of general-purpose computers and OA machines are now appearing. Simultaneously, terminals with multiple functions, or multifunction workstations are being introduced to save office space and to improve efficiency.

Impact of technology on jobs, work content and skills

Workers in EDP divisions and data-processing companies are particularly affected by the new computer and telecommunications technology. Operators' jobs, frequently involving shift work, can be simple and highly repetitive, with negative consequences. System engineers and programmers find that their working hours can be very long. At the same time, they face new types of psychological stress, such as having to keep up with technological developments, and worrying about major errors in large programmes. The practice in Japan of dispatching workers from computer manufacturing and data-processing companies to user firms for extended periods causes complicated personnel problems, as will be discussed later.

While there are few full-time operators of computer terminals or OA machines (fewer than 15 per cent of the workers who operate VDTs do this job more than four hours a day, according to the survey by the Ministry of Labour), some changes in job content have been observed. The survey reported simultaneous upgrading and downgrading of skills. For example,

133

while experience required for processing office work decreased, the machines also absorbed some routine tasks which enabled some workers to perform more interesting tasks, such as face-to-face contact with customers. The introduction of several kinds of OA machines or multi-functional workstations also enabled workers to carry out several simple tasks. A versatile semi-skilled clerical worker, a new type of white-collar worker, is emerging.

The tasks in operating OA machines are distributed in different ways. Sometimes a few workers, traditionally women workers, specialise in simple operating tasks. For example, it is often reported that, in sales branch offices, women office workers operate terminals to communicate the data of each salesman to head offices, while the salesmen are engaged solely in sales activities, armed with the information obtained from the systems.

A question of great interest is the extent to which a computerised information network will lead to the centralisation of authority and a decrease in discretionary power at the lower end of the hierarchy. A study by Shimada[1] showed that computerised information systems had not influenced upper-level staff, so that centralisation of decision-making power had not developed. Managers of head offices can get local information as quickly as they wish, but the workers at lower levels may also obtain company-wide information so far as it is allowed. However, a 1983 survey by the Ministry of International Trade and Industry (MITI) found that control of sales branches by head offices had been increased in 40 to 60 per cent of the firms in that (1) the objectives given to branches by head offices had become more detailed, (2) the frequency of checking the activities of branches by head offices had increased, (3) the directives addressed to branches had become more frequent and (4) the data sent to head offices from branches had increased.

Working conditions are changing with the application of the new technology in offices. According to the survey by the Ministry of Labour, 32 per cent of workers who were using OA machines reported that their work was easier than before, while 19 per cent felt their work had become harder. However, new occupational health problems are appearing. In particular, many workers complain of eyestrain after operating visual display terminals (VDTs) for long hours. In 1985, the Ministry of Labour published a concrete guide-line on various aspects of VDT use: ergonomic conditions, safety education, working hours and rest intervals, medical examination, and so on. Recently, newspapers have been interested in so-called "techno-stresses", the psychological stresses related to the new technology.

While there are common characteristics among sectors concerning technological change and its effects on workers, there are also differences. Banks have a long history of computerisation and have probably the most developed technology in the business world. The nature of work in commerce is different from that of offices. The technology applied in local government offices is still elementary but it is changing under a different social context. The data-processing industry is covered in this report because of the concentration of effects associated with technology on workers.

Advanced technology in the banking sector

Characteristics of the sector

There are several kinds of banks and financial institutions in Japan. These include city banks, regional banks, credit associations, agricultural co-operatives and government financial corporations. City banks, which number 13, will be the focus of this section as they have the most advanced computer and telecommunication systems.

The amount of deposits and loans handled by city banks has increased as Japan's economy has grown. In order to process the increasing office work, city banks have tried to computerise repetitive jobs to keep the workforce as small as possible. At the beginning of the 1960s, city banks introduced computers which worked as off-line batch systems to process data on expenditures and wages of their own employees and to collect statistical information.

On-line systems were then introduced in the middle of the 1960s in city banks. With these systems, major data on transactions at branch offices were processed in real time, that is the records of each customer account located in central computers were automatically adjusted at the time of deposits, withdrawals, and so on. Cash dispensers (CD) began to be used as terminals of these networks. In the first on-line systems, each type of bank activity, such as savings deposit or exchange, was managed separately. Difficulties in recruiting young female workers, and the need to improve the quality of customer services and to save on labour cost, prompted the innovations of this period.

A second group of on-line systems in city banks were introduced in the mid-1970s and are still in place. Business related to foreign exchange, loans and other services, which were not included in the first on-line sytems, were integrated. All individual customer accounts were combined under the customer's name, called CIF (consumer information file) or CMF (customer management file), a tool for learning a customer's financial position at a glance. Two inter-bank networks of cash dispensers were formed in 1980 and then linked together. The reasons for this system development were manifold: banks were supplying new types of services which needed computers; terminals at branches were becoming obsolete; and client firms were requesting improved services and more reliable operation without unexpected stoppages.

Since the oil crisis, the credit demand of enterprises has decreased. At the same time the costs related to deposits have increased. In this connection, bank managements were interested in reducing labour costs by means of further mechanisation, particularly through the introduction of improved terminals operated by bank employees and customers. Labour productivity in city banks increased remarkably: Bank A[2] estimated that the present level of labour productivity, that is, the number of transactions accomplished divided by the total number of employees, is five times higher than that of 20 years ago. The number of employees working at branch offices has decreased from 8,000 to 5,000 in these eight years, in spite of substantial increases in office work.

In a few years, city banks will start their third on-line systems as a strategic part of their business. "Cash management service" (CMS) and an extension of bank networks to firms ("firm banking") will develop further with these systems. The capacities of computers and terminals will be increased to new levels. International networks and information systems at the headquarters will be developed.

City banks have huge systems with large computers and nationwide networks. A good example is that of Bank B.

Bank B has a big computer centre in a 20-story building in downtown Tokyo. There are four sets of main computers installed for the on-line system. The first covers half of the terminals of each branch, with the second covering the other half. The third is a standby set of these two host computers. For example, if the first computer malfunctions, the third would take its place. The fourth computer is called a "system control and distribution computer". Its major functions are to control the two host computers and to distribute jobs that come into the system from outside, for instance from the banks' network, which connects cash dispensers (CDs) of all city banks.

Each branch office, more than 300 in number, has two terminal controllers, which are minicomputers, and various terminal devices. The total number of terminals is more than 10,000. Branch terminal computers are connected to host computers directly, or indirectly through relay stations. By this on-line real-time system, almost all transactions are

136

processed during office hours. Statistics for the use of branches are then processed and transmitted at night.

In 1986 Bank B introduced the third on-line system. In the new system, all necessary information is filed in data bases and processed for daily administrative work as well as for decision-making support in the head office. In addition, in 1982, the bank initiated an office automation campaign to encourage staff to use personal computers for appropriate tasks, such as some repetitive jobs, applications of statistical formulas and graphic presentations.

Industrial relations

Trade union leadership now promotes co-operation with management in city banks. In some categories of banks and financial institutions, the organised workers are divided into two groups with different orientations: the majority group with a co-operative attitude and the minority group critical toward management. There are often contrasting points of view between the two groups on various issues including the impact of new technology. To avoid conflicts, the management of city banks strives to foresee and solve problems before they occur. As an example, a manager of the office management division of a city bank stated that they had proposed their own ergonomic specifications to computer manufacturers when they ordered equipment.

Labour-management relations in city banks are conducted without outside observers. Employees of city banks are organised in company-wide unions; these unions are combined to form the Federation of City Bank Employees' Unions. There is a counterpart council of bank employers affiliated with the Japan Federation of Employers' Associations (Nikkeiren). Main collective relations exist at the company level. At Bank A, joint consultations are held at the head office about once a month. In addition, union representatives talk with managers informally. For example, with respect to the installation of a third on-line system, management explained its plans to the unions.

Joint consultations are held at the branch level in some banks. In a branch office of Bank B, the office manager talks with union representatives about working conditions once a month. A survey by the Saitama Prefectural Office on office automation shows that consultations are more frequent in the financial area and that workers are more positive on the introduction of OA machines compared with other industries.

The current on-line systems in city banks cover almost all customer banking transactions. When customers open savings accounts, detailed conditions of contracts are determined while the clerks are talking with the customers. Data are then entered into the systems through general-purpose terminals to make a new ledger file in the memory of the central computers. While customers wait, passbooks are prepared by the clerks. Bank A has developed a peripheral device called a LCT (low counter terminal) by which a passbook is issued by the time the consultation is finished. This means a traditional clerical task of writing with pen and ink is absorbed by the system, which thus frees clerks to expand their tasks of persuasion and consultation.

The procedure for funds transfer which is widely practised in Japan is automatic processing by the systems through automatic remittance terminals (ARs). A growing number of branches install ARs in their "automatic corners" where customers operate cash dispensers (CDs), auto-depositors (ADs) and automatic teller machines (ATMs). In a branch of Bank B located in downtown Tokyo, about 70 per cent of the customers who withdraw money and 50 per cent of those who make deposits use the automatic corner. The AR is used less often since it was introduced only recently.

On-line systems are used as a means of information on loans. The clerks who examine application documents can know the financial position of the applicant immediately. However, the decision of the bank to give a loan depends on the personal judgement of competent clerks and the approval of the branch manager or the manager of the head office.

On the whole, some of the traditional clerical jobs at the branch have been absorbed into the on-line systems. Tellers and clerks, who are mostly women, operate terminals during a substantial portion of their working hours. There are two major types of work, "counter" work and "second-line" office work, which consists of the routines for processing ongoing transactions. The current policy in city banks is to assign as many processing routines as possible to tellers doing "counter" work to reduce second-line office work. Tellers either work behind "high" counters, where requests regarding simple transactions such as deposits, withdrawals and funds transfers are made, or behind "low" counters where customers may consult with clerks or tellers on opening accounts, making time deposits, purchasing government bonds and so on.

The tellers who work behind the "high" counters use on-line teller machines (OTMs) or specialised terminals for tellers, and machines which make entries in passbooks automatically (STWs). Two devices which count money automatically, auto-cashiers (ACs) and coin cashiers (CCs), are being attached to OTMs. (These machine names are not totally standardised among banks). Operation of these terminal devices is not difficult to learn, and the scope of a teller's tasks is expanded to include the former second-line work and several categories of bank accounts. The number of categories of bank accounts that tellers can handle depends on their ability and experience.

At present, tellers behind high counters are engaged in repetitive work. For example, in one bank, 200 to 250 transactions are processed by a teller in a day, that is, from 9 a.m. to 3 p.m. except for the lunch interval. This means the average work cycle is less than 90 seconds. Tellers are now few in number: in a branch of Bank B with 65 employees, only five tellers work behind the high counter and two behind the low counter.

Tellers used to have the responsibility of reconciling their cash balance with the day's records, compiling statistical tables and processing related transactions after the office closed. Today, most of these jobs are unnecessary, and in any event, tellers are operating terminals of a system which stops working at the close of business. Between 3 p.m. and 5 p.m., they are assigned other subsidiary tasks such as putting bank slips and checks in order and counting them. They also help put money in order or engage in second-line office work, such as operating general-purpose terminals and checking various notices and inquiries regarding funds transfer.

General-purpose terminals are often used for low-counter work and for second-line work. With general-purpose terminals, operators select menus and items or enter data according to a set programme. To save labour costs related to the second-line work, city banks recently established local work-processing centres. One centre covers a few branch offices. The office jobs which have to be done mainly by hand are concentrated in these centres. A city bank with about 250 branches has 36 centres, with about 20 part-time workers and several bank employees in each centre. City banks have computer centres as cores of on-line systems. For example, Bank A with 15,000 employees has 180 staff members to operate its on-line system and 75 for batch processing. In addition, there are 60 to 70 operators dispatched from other companies carrying out computer support work. Other staff members engaged in check clearance, telex and other communications number more than 400.

In many industries the operation of the host computer is often contracted out, but the data filed in the computer centres are so important for banks that regular bank employees are responsible for their operation. In Bank B, operators, whose jobs are simple, are rotated at two-year intervals.

139

City banks have a large staff to develop software for the third on-line system. Bank A employs 400 system engineers and other technical staff. Those responsible for software development occasionally have to work long hours of overtime, especially when errors occur.

Computer centre employees in city banks tend to work in shifts. For example, in Bank B, there are three shifts, from 7.45 a.m. to 3.35 p.m., from 3 p.m. to 10 p.m., and from 9.45 p.m. to 5.45 p.m.

Because of the availability of information filed in the computer centres and the availability of personal computers, some bank employees will probably acquire new managerial skills. However, at this stage, opportunities for promotion have not been affected by computer and telecommunication technology on the whole.

Traditionally, men and women's jobs have been separated in banks as elsewhere. Banks have employed new female school graduates for the jobs of teller and second-line office worker or other subsidiary positions. The custom has been for women to resign within a few years to get married or have children. Recently, former female bank employees have been re-employed as part-time workers in local word-processing centres and as "lobby women" who, for example, assist customers on operating the terminals. The policy of lean staffing in banks appears to have encouraged female employees to expand the scope of their jobs. The Equal Employment Opportunity Law which came into force in April 1986 has influenced traditional practices. Women can now obtain similar positions and careers to men if they are able and willing to do so.

The percentage of female employees has been decreasing. This could be attributed mainly to computerisation of the jobs women traditionally hold. In 1976, women constituted approximately 47 per cent of city bank employees, according to city bank financial statements provided by the Federation of Bankers' Associations of Japan, whereas in 1984 they constituted approximately 38 per cent.

With few exceptions (managers, the inexperienced and, probably, staff members in charge of loans), male employees are engaged in outside duties relating to generating more business or attracting new clients. They are often obliged to work overtime by the nature of their outside jobs. They do not operate terminals to a significant extent. Generally, male employees have been rotated and promoted widely in their organisations.

Specific impact on VDT operators. A comparison of computer and telecommunication technology in city banks and other large corporations shows that network systems are far more developed in the banks, while other OA machines are less prevalent. It is expected that the impact of the new technology, if any, will be felt most by those workers who operate display terminals all day long or those who work in computer centres.

Judging from the 1983 survey by the Ministry of Labour, a relatively large number of workers operate terminals more than four hours a day in the financial sector, compared to other sectors. The percentage of firms in this sector which take special precautions for VDT operators – such as conducting medical examinations – was higher than in any other, according to the same survey. "Satisfied" workers who are using VDTs outnumbered those who expressed dissatisfaction. The most important reason for satisfaction was the reduction of overtime. However, about 60 per cent of VDT operators in banking, as in other fields, complained of eye strain, and 40 per cent complained of stiff shoulders. Occasionally, critical views have been expressed by minority union supporters concerning VDT work, shift work, high work intensity, overtime work, psychological stress, and so on. The survey by the Saitama Prefectural Office indicated that more than half of local managers recognised the need for improved health protection.

Technological and organisational design options

Substantive aspect. City banks have office management divisions which analyse the work at branch offices and standardise the forms of documents and business procedures. They apply industrial engineering techniques, based on the assumption that some organisational units resemble a factory. According to one interviewee, all jobs are divided into standardised infinitesimal units, then the standard time required to perform the units is measured. These units are then combined to form a task to be done in a specific time. Various tasks are distributed among employees. The introduction of new machines means that new units and tasks are created and some old ones are eliminated. Clearly, management has options for assigning tasks to individual workers or to groups of workers.

Before computerisation there were two types of work flow at branch offices: one organised by categories of account and another by functions or occupations of employees, that is tellers, machine operators and assistants. The limited capacity of the machines as well as managerial policies were the basis of this differentiation. With the current on-line systems, tasks of tellers generally cover several categories of account and second-line office work. Individual tellers are encouraged to master as many tasks as possible. A survey by Ningen Noryoku Kaihatsu Senta (Centre for the Development of Human Abilities) in 1983 revealed that 70 per cent of city banks had policies to expand the scope of tasks assigned to individual workers, after the introduction of cash dispensers and

141

terminals. Relationships between individual employees and tasks are flexible, as the employees working in an office will relieve tellers from work at any time depending on circumstances. The current organisation at the branch office is, therefore, based on groups. Another indication that assignment of tasks is related to groups has been the introduction of quality circles.

The current on-line systems are highly centralised from a technical viewpoint, but this does not necessarily mean that decision-making is centralised. However, the previously mentioned survey by MITI showed that head offices tended to increase their control over branch offices through more detailed specification of objectives, more frequent checking and requests for reports.

Banks also practise a sort of management by objectives in which head offices determine detailed quantitative standards in each field of business after consultations with branch managers. This management practice was unrelated originally to the technological systems, but obviously these systems can work as a main tool to facilitate this practice.

At branch level, access to general-purpose terminals is gained by using a key which identifies a user. One purpose of this procedure is to do an internal audit, but personal performance or correctness of operations might also be measured. Employee ratings are widely used in Japanese firms, including banks, as a means of personnel management. There is always a possibility that records of terminal operations will be used to appraise the performance of operators. In fact, a branch manager said that he had referred to the records of individual operators which indicated the number of all cases handled as well as errors corrected. These records are taken as objective indicators of performance or accuracy of employees for this manager. The methodology and results of employee ratings can be a subject of labour-management consultation or informal grievance handling in some companies, although this kind of information in city banks is not revealed to outside observers. Human organisations co-existing with technical systems might be subject to centralised control, if appropriate safeguards are not provided.

Procedural aspect. In Bank B a project team for office automation was formed, probably to listen to the views and needs of each division, to create a positive attitude toward the project and to reach consensus. As previously explained, when banks wish to introduce a new system or equipment, the bank management decides on a plan first and then explains the plan to its union. A quality circle is one of the routes through which ordinary employees express their opinions concerning their work. Their proposals might be considered by the office management division in developing standard procedures.

Future perspectives

Sophisticated international networks will contribute to bringing higher returns in funds management. Through firm banking, banks will provide new services in exchange for charges. The nature of the new systems is not new, however. Since one of the objectives of the new systems is to minimise labour costs, it is expected that there will be curtailed employment in city banks.

It is possible that the new systems may influence workers in other industries as networks are connected with outside firms. For example, firm banking could release workers in other firms from the repetitive job of recording incoming and outgoing money.

Bank management is cautious about the ill effects of VDTs, but complaints still remain. This is an urgent problem to be solved.

The current technological systems provide possibilities for centralised control, but whether or not they are realised will depend on managerial policies.

Advanced technology in wholesale and retail trade

Characteristics of the sector

The wholesale and retail trades have been providing numerous opportunities for employment in Japan since the first oil crisis in 1973. The majority of workers are employed as family owners and family workers or as employees of small retail shops. The relative importance of the traditional retail trade has decreased gradually as large, modern distributive firms have emerged.

A Japanese-style department store deals in all sorts of goods handled by specialty stores, in addition to food. There are 360 department stores in Japan; their share in total retail sales is less than 10 per cent. Although department stores have enjoyed a reputation for quality goods and the trust of customers, their traditional way of doing business is at a crossroads, as new types of retailing have been emerging. Department stores were the first among commercial firms to experiment with POS (point-of-sale) systems.

The Japanese-style supermarket is a self-service store dealing mostly in food. A self-service store mainly dealing in clothes is called a "superstore". Large companies of both categories have many branches in the suburban shopping areas or other busy places not far from railway stations. These firms are often members of the Japan Chain Stores Association. Large self-service stores with more than 50 employees number nearly 1,900 and have sales almost the equivalent of those of department stores in recent years. Since they appeared, their growth in sales has been remarkable, especially in the period of high economic growth, but now the period of rapid expansion seems to be over.

Consumer behaviour in Japan is believed to have changed in recent years. Buyers now attach more importance to the high quality of goods than to cost, especially for goods that they buy occasionally. At the same time, they prefer cheaper items for daily necessities. Self-service stores, as well as specialty stores, have to adjust themselves to the current preferences of consumers, by providing a variety of items in small volume. POS can play an important role in this connection.

The channels of distribution in Japan are very complicated. The total number of wholesale establishments is approximately 400,000. Average wholesalers have more employees than average retailers. Trading companies, large or small, are also classified in the wholesale trade. It is estimated that the nine general trading companies known as *Sogo shosha* deal with nearly half of Japan's exports and more than 60 per cent of her imports. Large companies in the wholesale trade, especially general trading companies, have computerised information systems, and they are promoting office automation.

Main types of advanced technology

Commerce has the largest number of computers of all sectors. According to statistics of the MITI, there were 131,000 computers in place in July 1983, of which 60,000 or 45 per cent belonged to the wholesale and retail trades. However, the average price of computers in this sector is the lowest. This indicates that average wholesalers and large retailing firms have introduced office computers more widely than large, general-purpose computers. For example, a general trading company with 6,000 employees has 450 display terminals and 110 printers linked to one medium-sized and two large-sized computers. The major function of the system is to process data on transactions, such as contracts, and the flow of commodities and money. Like other general trading companies, this company has approximately one dozen divisions, one of which deals in computers and communication equipment. About ten office computers are installed to meet the data-processing needs of specific divisions. This company is now engaged in developing a telecommunication network which connects computers and terminals, and is promoting OA to

144

minimise repetitive work and to obtain useful information for management from the daily transaction data.

POS is not as developed in Japan as in other industrialised countries (see figure 2). According to a survey by MITI, about one-third of the department stores and chain stores, and one-quarter of the specialty stores had POS terminals in 1982. If the companies which were considering introducing them are included, the figure rises to 60 or 70 per cent. POS is spreading from department stores to self-service stores and from large enterprises to smaller ones. According to the survey by MITI, the purposes of introducing POS are to manage individual commodity items or store sections and to save human resources. It is particularly important for department stores to get information on customers in relation to payment by credit cards, which are being used increasingly. In order to manage individual items effectively, data input at POS terminals

Figure 2   Point-of-sales (POS) systems in shops

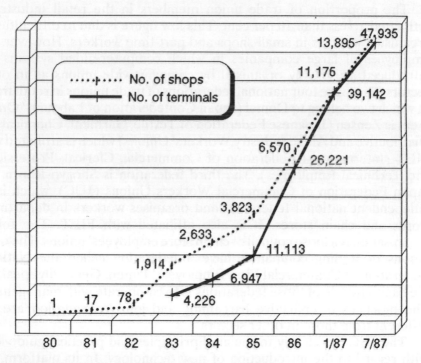

Source: *Nikkei OA Neuken* (Nikkei's OA Yearbook), 1988.

is used in controlling stock and ordering. This is practised in most speciality stores and 60 per cent of chain stores using POS terminals. A survey by the Japan Chain Stores Association indicates that self-service stores are also eager to use POS terminals.

A characteristic POS plan is an on-line system with a host computer installed at the headquarters, store controllers (minicomputers) at stores and POS terminals at check-out counters. The scanners attached to POS terminals read "bar codes" or OCR (optical character recognition) letters automatically to put data into the system. In some specialty stores and department stores, data are entered by using keys, depending on the categories of commodities.

The low diffusion rate of source marking, that is, printing of bar codes by manufacturers or suppliers, and the high costs of introducing the equipment in comparison with the wages of part-time cashiers, are major reasons why POS systems have not been widely used in Japan.

Industrial relations

The proportion of trade union members in the retail industry is estimated at less than 10 per cent. This low figure is due to difficulties in organising workers in small shops and part-time workers. However, the employees of large companies in which computer-aided systems are introduced are mostly organised by company-wide unions as in other sectors. There are four national federations of trade unions in retail trade, of which two belong to Domei (Japan Confederation of Labour).[3] One of them is Zensen (Japanese Federation of Textile, Garment, Chemical and Distributive and Allied Industry Workers' Unions) which is affiliated with FIET (International Federation of Commercial, Clerical, Professional and Technical Employees). The third federation is Shogyo-Roren, the Japan Federation of Commercial Workers Unions (JUC), which is an independent national federation and organises workers in department stores and chain stores. It is also affiliated with FIET. The fourth organisation is a loose council of chain store employees' unions. The trade unions of trading companies have a federation called the National Federation of Commercial Firm Employees' Union. Generally speaking, the basic attitude of those federations is to co-operate with management. The practices of collective bargaining and joint consultation are not different from those in other sectors.

The JUC has clearly formulated principles and practical guide-lines with regard to the introduction of new technology. In its platform, the JUC states that it promotes productivity if workers share in the resulting benefits. A JUC pamphlet on union participation in management asserts that the source of workers' welfare is the enterprise employing them, and a union has to exert its own efforts to increase the profitability of the enterprise. Based on this principle, member unions are to accept new technology with due precautions for security of employment, the protection of working conditions, and so on. For the Federation, prior consultation at the enterprise level is important from a procedural viewpoint.

Changes in jobs and skills

The employment conditions of computer workers in retailing are in general similar to those in other sectors. However, there are slight differences in that the development of software is subcontracted less frequently, and a substantial number of keypunchers are still employed in a few department stores.

Some studies show that the introduction of POS terminals in department stores seem to have had little influence on the jobs of sales assistants, who more or less specialise by categories of goods or sections of the store. At Department Store X, the first to introduce POS, the skills required to operate POS terminals are nearly similar to those of handling the former cash registers. Operation of the terminals is a minor part of the tasks of the group or of individual sales assistants in terms of both the skills and the time required. The practice of allowing a group of sales assistants (including part-time workers) under a section supervisor to decide their respective tasks has not changed. The present POS system makes it easy for sales assistants to respond immediately to customer inquiries and to concentrate more on selling.

A case study on POS by Zensen in 1982 showed that the tasks of sales assistants had changed a little. Some tasks related to proper maintenance of stock and ordering were taken over by the system, but the reading of printed data was added to other tasks. More time was spent with customers. Jobs at store offices and head offices were also influenced by the new system. Paperwork and manual calculation were replaced by the operation of display terminals. It is expected that the analysis of information processed by the system would become an important skill of the staff responsible for planning, purchasing, store management, and so on. As source marking was not widely done, in-store marking jobs increased.

There are no comprehensive surveys on the division of labour in self-service stores, but usually cashiers specialise in the tasks that their name denotes. Regular employees are transferred and promoted from one job to another after a few years of service. Some important jobs, such as handling money or ordering goods, are assigned to regular employees. However, women part-time women workers as well as student temporary workers are engaged in various jobs in each store. According to a survey by Zensen, part-time workers and regular employees are working side by side at check-out counters. However, with the widespread introduction of POS terminals, it is expected that regular employees will be transferred to other sections and will be replaced by part-time employees.

Operating POS terminals is considered simpler than using electronic cash registers (ECRs). A supermarket manager indicated that the initial training period for newly hired cashiers had decreased probably from three days to one day. Zensen found that average initial training periods for newly hired employees, some of whom became cashiers, is about a week. In this period, they are taught how commodities are classified and how to operate ECRs or POS terminals, in addition to other subjects such as the structure of the company, work rules and working conditions.

A few self-service stores pay a small allowance to cashiers responsible for money. It is uncertain if the POS system will affect this practice.

Each self-service store has several shifts and working schedules to match fluctuations in sales and the preferences of part-time workers. It seems that so far these working schedules are not related to any attempt to regulate the working hours of POS terminal workers.

Corresponding to the wide diffusion of computers in this sector, more workers spend longer hours relating to computerised systems, compared with other sectors. About 20 per cent of the workers who use general-purpose computers work more than six hours a day, and approximately 10 to 15 per cent of the workers who operate on-line terminals or VDTs work more than four hours.

According to a 1983 survey of the Ministry of Labour, more than 60 per cent of workers who operated VDTs complained of eye strain, and about 50 per cent of stiff shoulders. A JUC survey in 1983 revealed 81 per cent of union members of EDP divisions had eye difficulties "often" or "occasionally". In spite of these complaints, the number of workers operating OA machines who reported that their work was easier than before exceeded those who reported otherwise. The JUC survey also showed that 70 per cent of the workers questioned were "satisfied" or "rather satisfied" with their jobs. Major causes of dissatisfaction were related to the work itself in the organisation. Among the reasons given were the lack of understanding within the company of the significance of their jobs, poor scheduling of work, excessive overtime work, poor work environment and mental stress.

Technological and organisational design options

Substantive aspect. The JUC survey on EDP divisions classified workers by major types of jobs. The jobs of programmers, operators, system engineers and service engineers (those mainly responsible for maintenance of hardware) were specifically designated. Twelve per cent of the respondents performed all four of these jobs. This reflects the fact that EDP tasks are allocated to the division as an organisational unit and are distributed among its members fluidly. In EDP divisions, such tasks as keypunching, communicating with other sections, and consulting with and training the staff of user departments are likewise assigned fluidly.

A high level of computer technology knowledge is required to perform EDP work. According to a department store manager and a superstore manager, the length of service in their EDP divisions was longer than in other divisions because of the technical knowledge required. At the same time, however, the status of the EDP staffs and the managers has not always been high.

As previously stated, all section members in Department Store X used POS terminals in principle, while in self-service stores cashiers specialised in operating them. This difference had been established before POS systems started. Therefore, the allocation of tasks among workers is likely to be independent from the technological system.

At Superstore Company Y, a POS system with 8,000 terminals was introduced. This was a big event, as the total number of POS terminals of all member companies of the Japan Chain Stores Association was 13,000 in 1984. In an interview with the management, we were told that the company had centralised its decision-making several years before the decision to introduce POS terminals was made. As a result of this centralisation of decision-making, the purchasing function, which formerly belonged to store managers, was placed in the hands of buyers at the head office. Store managers are also directed by corporate supervisors. The store managers' major functions now relate to the administration of sales activities and personnel, including the recruitment of part-time workers. The POS system of this company is a centralised information system from a technological point of view. It has not changed the distribution of decision-making power anew, but supports the centralised decision-making previously established by providing the necessary information instantly. It provides a means to evaluate the efficiency of employees and managers. Thus, POS systems may work as a tool to facilitate centralised or decentralised personnel management.

In Company Y, a "clock-in system" was introduced before the start of the POS system. This computerised system is used for recording attendance and for calculating pay. The attendance data of 36,000 workers of 140 establishments in various shifts are processed by the system. The corporate personnel department as well as store managers have access to these personnel records at any time. This system too can work as a tool for centralised personnel management aside from enabling store managers to adjust the daily schedules of workers to meet various requirements.

Procedural aspect. There are no remarkable differences, compared with other sectors, in the procedural aspect of introducing the new technology. The POS manual of the Japan Chain Stores Association recommends forming project teams. A basic plan is to be formulated by a development team. A working party will translate this plan into a concrete programme and promote it. A design committee of the EDP division will design the system and develop the software.

Trade unions do not usually participate in the project teams established to develop computerised systems or to promote office automation, but are consulted at a later stage of planning. The importance of joint consultation on new technology is widely accepted retailing sector, but many unions are informed only after the plans for new technology have been completed. Therefore, one of the targets of trade unions with respect to new technology is to have consultations at the formative planning stage. The technology committee of the JUC recommends that member unions form a joint planning committee if necessary. In accordance with this guide-line, representatives of the employees' union of Self-service Store Z joined a planning committee as well as a working party to introduce a POS system. However, this is a rather exceptional case of participation. Some shop-floor workers consider the introduction of a POS system as a natural improvement. Therefore, in spite of the clauses on joint consultation in labour-management agreements, relatively "minor" changes, such as the introduction of word processors, might not come to the attention of union representatives.

Future perspectives

As new technology develops in the wholesale and retail trade, new types of commerce such as "home shopping", are emerging. The data on customers' attributes, tastes, financial positions, records of purchase, and so on, are filed and processed to anticipate their demands. Various types of telecommunication networks among firms are also rapidly developing. A few firms or groups of firms are pioneering in these areas. At this stage, it is difficult to foresee the social impact of these emerging changes.

150

POS is a specific application of the new technology in this sector. This system is expected to be used in more large-scale retail firms. POS is essentially an information system and the distribution of decision-making power is independent from the system in any given firm. However, it will be necessary for intermediary wholesalers, manufacturers and delivery services to respond quickly to orders communicated through an inter-firm network. The mode of decision-making in these firms might be influenced.

Advanced technology in local governments

Characteristics of the sector

There are two levels of local government, with autonomy guaranteed by the Japanese Constitution. At present there are 47 prefectures and about 3,300 municipalities (cities, towns and villages). The administrators (governors, mayors or heads) and assembly members of these bodies are elected by the residents. Municipalities are defined as basic localities, while prefectures deal with the administration of matters covering wide areas such as co-ordination among municipalities, and so on. Municipalities are responsible for matters which relate to the day-to-day life of an average resident, such as family registration, resident registration, certification of registered seals which are used for important private contracts, and records involving National Health Insurance and National Pension Insurance, primary and junior high school education, resident and fixed property taxes, public health and social welfare. Therefore, ordinary citizens come into contact with the offices of municipalities more often than those of prefectures. Prefectural offices have similar types of transactions in spite of less frequent contacts with residents. In a few fields of prefectural administration, such as taxes, the coverage of the whole prefectural population is necessary.

During the period of high economic growth in Japan, the accompanying geographical redistribution of the population caused financial difficulties for depopulated towns and villages as well as for some cities with a large influx of population. Since the high economic growth ended with the oil crisis in 1973, local governments have been faced with serious financial difficulties: tax revenues have not increased much while administrative, welfare and other expenditures have tended to escalate rapidly. Currently, local governments are trying to cut expenditures in line with nation-wide administrative and financial reform. Some administrators of local governments have been interested in computerisation to

151

keep the workforce at a minimum and, possibly, to put the resulting surplus staff in the services which need to be strengthened. The number of local government employees increased in the 1960s and 1970s, exceeding 3 million.

The autonomy of local government has been a focus of social concern throughout the four decades of the postwar period. A large number of national laws, subsidies and administrative guide-lines determine or influence the responsibilities and actions of local governments in various ways and thus the scope of real autonomy of local government is limited.

The supporters of local autonomy are vigilant lest the recent applications of computer and telecommunication technology should cause further deterioration of local self-government. They are also concerned with how to protect the privacy of residents whose personal data are filed in the computerised system. Personal data have been recorded at several sections of municipal or prefectural offices for particular official uses, and the officials in charge are expected to maintain confidentiality. However, if scattered data are gathered to establish a computerised personal file for each individual resident or family, without careful protective measures, such information might easily be used by anybody.

Applications of advanced technology

In the administration of local government, the application of computer and telecommunication technology, although not developed to the extent it is in private industry, is accelerating.

General-purpose computers were first used to process massive routine office work involving matters such as taxation, social insurance and wages. In the early 1960s a few large cities and prefectures began to introduce computers. Since then the use of computers has spread to other local governments and various categories of administrative jobs. At present, all prefectures have installed computers, including office computers, and 96 per cent of the municipalities are also using them. Figure 3 shows the number of municipalities which introduced computers for themselves or jointly with other municipalities, and the number who contract out their work to data-processing firms. In prefectures, wages, taxation, statistics and other massive office work are processed by computers. Computers are also used by most of the prefectures in planning and accounting. In municipalities the work on taxation and National Health Insurance premiums is very often processed by computers. In small towns and villages, however, these jobs can be efficiently handled by traditional means.

152

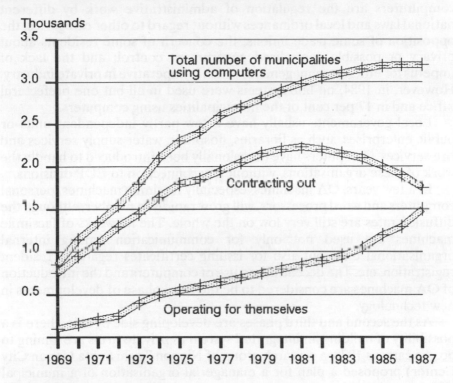

Figure 3   Number of municipalities which use computers

Thousands

Total number of municipalities
using computers

Contracting out

Operating for themselves

1969 1971 1973 1975 1977 1979 1981 1983 1985 1987

Source: Ministry of Home Affairs.

At first, computers were used on a batch-processing basis to replace repetitive manual work, without considering relationships between categories of administrative work to be processed. Local government employees have nicknamed the computers used in this way "big abacuses". However, as the second phase of the application of new technology, some local governments began to use a computer as a nucleus of an information system rather than as a big abacus. The on-line system and data bases are examples of new developments. In addition to these two developments, Chinese characters can now be used for the input and output of data while only *kana* (the Japanese syllabary) was used before. This is important, for public offices, as individual persons are identified by names written in Chinese characters. These three recent developments in this sector, which are taken for granted in other sectors, are called "the advanced uses of computers" by local government employees.

153

Obstacles to introducing data-base systems and advanced uses of computurers are the regulation of administrative work by different national laws and local ordinances without regard to other categories; the opposition of some trade unions; the concern of some residents about privacy or possible centralised government control; and the lack of impetus for efficient management, which is imperative in private industry. However, in 1984, on-line systems were used in all but one prefectural office and in 17 per cent of the municipalities using computers.

Local governments usually have a few partly independent units or public enterprises, such as libraries, hospitals, water supply services and fire services. Computers have occasionally been introduced to handle the work of these organisations, without any connection to EDP divisions.

In a few years, OA machines, especially facsimile machines, personal computers and word processors, will grow rapidly in number, although the diffusion rates are still very low on the whole. The networks of facsimile machines are used not only for communication among internal organisational units but also for issuing certificates regarding resident registration, etc. The decentralised use of computers and the introduction of OA machines are considered to be the third phase of developments in new technology.

As the second and third phases are developing side by side, there is a possibility of building an integrated system as private firms are aiming to do. As early as 1978, a research group of Nippon Toshi Senta (Japan City Center) proposed a plan for a managerial organisation of a municipal office supported by a computerised network. This plan was called the Municipal Total Information System (MTIS). This total system is composed of three subsystems: the residents' information system concerning welfare, education, public health, medical care, taxation, elections, and so on; the internal management information system concerning personnel management, accounting, planning, recording, and so on; and the environmental information system concerning urban planning, environmental protection, traffic, disaster prevention, adult education, industries and commerce, and so on. The report emphasises that an institutional organisation had to change in such a way as to match the integrated computerised system with appropriate data bases in place of the division of jobs by administrative fields. It also provides a basic framework on which local governments may base their own plans if they wish to utilise fully computer and telecommunication technology. But so far no local government has fully implemented this kind of plan.

In spite of the lag in the application of new technology in this sector, some administrators of prefectures and large cities are now interested in the so-called "new media" administration which includes policies concerning two-way communication between local governments and residents and the application of new communication tools to administration and services in specific fields. At present, the new media which have practical meaning in terms of local government are probably CATV (cable TV), CAPTAIN (videotext) and VRS (video response system). Many local governments have formed study groups or project teams on this subject.

Industrial relations

Labour relations of ordinary local government employees are regulated by two different laws. The Local Public Service Law applies to civil servants employed in ordinary administrative organisations, while the Local Public Enterprise Labour Relations Law applies to employees of local public enterprises, such as transportation or water supply services. According to the Local Public Service Law, unions of local government employees can discuss collectively with management but they cannot enter into collective agreements, except on issues which are covered in local ordinances. For example, salaries and other employment conditions are stipulated by ordinances. In prefectures and certain specified large cities, local personnel committees make recommendations on the revision of salary scales and employment conditions, and the assemblies deliberate on the recommendations to enact ordinances on the issues. Strikes are prohibited for both categories of local government employees. Due to the above and other restrictions, the unions of ordinary local civil servants have difficulties in pressing their demands.

The unions of workers employed by local public enterprises have the right to bargain collectively and enter into collective agreements compatible with ordinances. According to the law, wages have to be determined by ordinances but other employment conditions, including salary levels, are open to bargaining. However, in practice, most working conditions of the workers are stipulated by ordinances. In this field, trade unions and management first reach agreement and then the administrators propose the revision of the relevant ordinances to the assemblies. In many cases, the two categories of local government employees join together to form a trade union. Occasionally, councils of workers employed by local public enterprises are formed. They also sometimes unite to form their own unions and these unions then organise national federations.

The employees of local governments often form a local union which has complete autonomy. These local unions then join a federation. The

155

representative national federation is the All-Japan Prefectural and Municipal Workers' Union (Jichiro) which is affiliated with Sohyo.

Formal collective relations exist between local government employees and the corresponding local government management. The basic employment conditions of local government employees are determined through a complicated process under the supervision of the national Government. The issues on employment and working conditions related to the introduction of new systems or OA machines are handled between top-level union representatives and local government officials. The two laws mentioned previously exclude administrative and managerial matters from collective bargaining. Thus the introduction of new systems or OA machines itself is a managerial prerogative; but detailed conditions with regard to these innovations may be discussed at the level of the workplace.

In the early 1970s, Jichiro adopted three principles on computers or information. The first principle concerns the use of computers for peaceful purposes and for the improvement of the standard of living. The second relates to the democratic control of data processing, which implies the influence of workers in the introduction and management of the equipment and the protection of workers from alienating jobs. The third concerns protecting the privacy of residents. However, some people indicated that it was not clear whether these three principles were meant to prevent the introduction of computerised systems or whether they were the minimum union standards on which these systems were to be introduced. It is perhaps important to note that in the late 1970s there were some unionists who proposed to fight to stop the introduction of computerised systems.

They considered union activities concerning advance joint consultations and democratic control of work systems as ineffective. At its general meeting in 1979, Jichiro adopted a policy to prevent the advanced uses of computers. This official policy was not abandoned, at least through 1984 and 1985, in spite of the widespread use of computers. At its general meeting in 1984, Jichiro developed guide-lines which recommend the following to its members: (1) to oppose any attempt to reduce the workforce or transfer workers due to the introduction of computers or OA machines without collective agree- ments; (2) to repel similar attempts unless agreements are reached in writing; (3) to demand improvements in working conditions in EDP sections and workplaces where OA machines are used; (4) to prohibit contracting out of jobs in principle; (5) to disallow use of programmes and systems which are beyond the control of local government employees; and (6) to refuse to connect OA machines with host computers in principle.

156

With regard to the application of new technology, the policies of individual local government unions and the developments in union-management relations are varied. In one medium-sized city the administrator succeeded in introducing a computerised system without any resistance from the militant union leaders, while in another city the union was somewhat co-operative with management as the union members welcomed computerisation.

In ward office A,[4] a computer was first introduced in 1967. In 1976, an on-line system having a data base of combined residents' records in *kana* was introduced. Approximately every five years the ward office updated its medium-term plans on the mechanisation of office work. In the fifth plan, one of the important objectives is to install a new on-line system with an extended data base of residents' records in Chinese characters. The ward management planned to put the terminals of this on-line system at administrative service centres which were to replace branch offices. An administrative service centre is a combined facility including a meeting room, a children's nursery and a day-care centre for the aged.

The trade union disputed the installation of the on-line system and the establishment of administrative service centers. When a project team was formed by the ward in 1981, the union decided to oppose the plan but allowed union representatives to attend the team meeting as observers. The union embarked on various activities to substantiate its position and submitted its views and official demands to the administrator in August 1983. In objecting to the establishment of the administrative service centre, the union principally argued that working conditions would deteriorate and that the new system would be inconvenient for the residents.

The management categorically refused the union demands on the plan itself, and stuck to provisions on management prerogatives. The union tried to gain support from the residents and the assembly members. In December 1983, at the third session of collective bargaining, both parties reached an agreement on prior joint consultation on working conditions. After this basic agreement was reached, there were detailed consultations between the parties. The union submitted a series of demands, such as increasing the number of workers or regulating overtime in the EDP section. The union also concerned itself with health problems related to VDT work. At the request of the ward an ergonomic and industrial hygiene study was undertaken by the Institute for Science of Labour. In September 1984 a guide-line on VDT work was published by the head of the ward. The new on-line system started in June 1985, after various issues were resolved.

If we take the total number of local governments and their employees into consideration, it seems that computers and OA machines are not widely used. According to statistics of the Ministry of Home Affairs, less than 10,000 local civil servants were working in EDP sections in 1984. There were 47,000 computers, 4,000 personal computers and 2,000 word processors in prefectures and municipalities.

The staff of EDP divisions in local governments are generally not highly specialised. This could be attributed to the fact that the transfer of staff to and from EDP divisions is fairly common and that, in many cases, each worker has two or more computer-related tasks. However, sections with voluminous, standardised paperwork may have partly specialised operators of terminals or personal computers. In other cases, terminals of host computers and other OA machines including word processors are used occasionally by a wide circle of workers. For the sake of efficiency, OA specialists have recommended setting up word-processing centres for large-volume jobs. But in reality, several prefectural offices have dissolved such centres because of the difficulties in keeping the flow of work constant.

A survey by Associate Professor Kainuma in 1985[5] on the working conditions and attitudes of VDT operators of city B, which is noted for its advanced computerised system, showed 4.5 per cent of the operators worked an average of more than four hours a day on VDUs. A 1983 Jichiro survey (of which the sampling method is unknown) of about 600 VDT operators reported a much higher figure and pointed out that the operating hours are much longer in busy seasons. It cannot be denied that there are a few clerks who specialise in VDT jobs and who are occasionally obliged to work long hours. However, the majority of workers who operate computer terminals and OA machines spend only part of their working hours on such jobs.

The Jichiro survey reported that 95 per cent of VDT operators performed other office tasks such as ordinary desk work, receiving visitors, checking output data, and so on. The survey also showed that the major types of VDT work were data input, retrieval and dialogue-type tasks, and that female workers were engaged in the first two types more often than male workers.

The survey by Kainuma revealed that more than half of the female VDT operators thought their jobs were repetitive and required little discretion but that their work pace was not always strictly controlled. But some employees in the head office of city B felt that the work processed by VDTs required some degree of discretion. According to a 1984 opinion survey by Jichiro, local civil servants who were working in EDP sections or using word processors tended to feel that they had opportunities to develop their abilities while working.

Generally speaking, the practice of transferring staff between EDP sections and other sections is fairly common in local governments. However, the duration of service of the workers in computer-related jobs is likely to be longer than that of other workers.

The wages and overtime work in the sections with computerised systems are worth noting. The Jichiro opinion survey revealed that a substantial number of male and female workers in EDP sections and male workers using computerised systems felt that their wages did not match their jobs. This is a difficult problem because the salaries of local government employees are not specifically determined by the nature of their jobs. The survey also reported long overtime work in EDP sections because of the shortage of staff and frequent changes in software specifications.

Some jobs in EDP sections – software development, operation of main computers and keypunching – are frequently contracted out because of the difficulties in personnel management, in particular in respect of shift work, lack of qualified workers and the monotonous nature of the jobs.

According to the opinion survey by Jichiro, the proportion of union members who felt their jobs worthwhile was very high among EDP workers. On the other hand, the corresponding figure for female workers who were operating terminals was low, with even more dissatisfaction among keypunchers in EDP sections. The male workers who were operating terminals came between the above two groups. In the survey by Kainuma, the majority of terminal operators were positive about their jobs, but felt that the working environment, task management and health protection should be improved.

In spite of their generally positive attitudes, computer terminal operators are faced with new health problems. According to the Jichiro survey in 1983 nearly one-half of VDT operators reported problems with their eyes, and doctors diagnosed approximately 10 per cent of these cases as eye strain. The survey detected a series of physical health complaints similar to those in other sectors. A few member unions of Jichiro arrived at an agreement with local government administrators on working conditions with respect to VDTs. Jichiro formulated guide-lines on this issue at the end of August 1985.

Substantive aspect. Like large private firms, local governments have the lifetime employment practice where young people are employed for unspecified jobs as local civil servants, then transferred among various divisions. Jobs are classified by divisions, sections and subsections, and so on, and individual workers, particularly those at lower levels, are expected to behave as members of their groups These practices have not really changed with the application of new technology.

Kainuma points out that the introduction of computerised networks tends to bring about the centralisation of decision-making and the separation of the functions of planning and executing, as well as the polarisation of workers. In practice, the distribution of decision-making power in local government offices is complicated, although it might be clarified in the course of the introduction of each computerised system. For the time being, OA machines are introduced into organisational units without major changes in the existing distribution of authority.

Procedural aspect. Each local government stands at a different stage of new technology application, due mainly to differences in the policies of administrators. Teams of middle management which deal with "new media administration" or office automation are presently working in many prefectures and cities. The managers in charge of EDP sections often play important roles in relation to the work of these teams.

In recent years some local governments have been promoting quality circles (which are concerned with quality and the pursuit of perfection), in addition to suggestion schemes, to improve the efficiency of office work and the quality of services.

The attitudes of trade unions in this sector generally contrast with those in private industry. The unions tend to rely on collective bargaining rather than on joint consultation to achieve their objectives. Judging from the few cases referred to previously, trade unions are definitely playing an important role in determining how the new technology is actually used.

Future perspectives

Application of new technology in local governments is accelerating and the tendency will continue in the near future, as they have to follow outside technological and managerial developments. Financial difficulties and increasing demand for administrative services are promoting the advanced uses of computerised systems, in spite of some union resistance.

Although it is difficult to forecast the long-term effects of computerised networks on the nature of work, repetitive tasks such as data input will probably remain. Efforts of management to curtail labour costs may result in a heavier work load. However, if VDT use is properly regulated, many workers would continue to welcome its introduction since it makes work easier and provides challenging opportunities to learn new skills and new jobs.

Advanced technology in the data processing industry

Characteristics of the sector

The growth of the data-processing industry in Japan has been remarkable, with a turnover in 1984 five times that in 1975. The industry has responded to the needs of business and society as the use of computers has become widespread.

The Industry is composed of (1) the software business, consisting of a group of software houses mainly engaged in the development of computer programmes; (2) data-processing services, provided both within the service companies and by workers dispatched from them; (3) information (or data-base) service companies which provide information retrieval services; and (4) other information services.

The average size of firms in this sector is small, with 53.6 per cent of the employees in 1984 working in companies with less than 30 employees. Statistics from MITI show that 40 per cent of the firms do not have their own computers.

So far, the market for software for general use has not developed in Japan except for personal computers. The main activity of software houses is to participate in software development projects for mainframe general-purpose computers.

When computers were expensive, firms contracted out their data-processing work. When the prices came down relative to performance, firms preferred to do it themselves. On the other hand, some companies have started to contract out the operation of their computers to cut expenditures and avoid personnel problems such as shift work and low morale.

Data-base services have emerged, but they are at an early stage. About 900 data bases of 75 companies were registered at MITI in 1984. The majority of these companies sell data-base services as a sideline. CAPTAIN (Character and Pattern Telephone Access Information

Network), the videotext in Japan, began its service in November 1984 and will contribute to the development of data-base services.

Computer technology influences the software, which may in turn influence the internal organisation and employment conditions of the firms. Considering this linkage, changes in computer technology and organisation of work are worth noting.

First of all, with the technology developing rapidly, companies have found business opportunities by providing consultancy services on technical matters, dispatching specialists to users, developing programmes or establishing new services. As an example, computer technology is currently being connected with telecommunication technology, and engineers with expertise in both fields are needed. Remote computing service (RCS) and value added network (VAN) services are some of the new fields in the business.

Secondly, peripheral equipment has a direct impact on work. The method of entering data has changed from punching cards to optical character recognition (OCR) processing or direct operation of keyboards at terminals. The operation of general-purpose computers is being automated and the jobs of operators are becoming simpler.

Thirdly, specialised computers and software for the development of new programmes are being introduced. This will also affect the employment conditions of workers in this area.

Industrial relations

Union-management relations are based on the relationship between individual workers and management, particularly in small firms. Workers are more specialised in their jobs than they are in other industries where regular workers are transferred from one job to another within the firm under the lifetime employment system.

The organisation rate by trade unions in this sector is low. The practice of dispatching employees to different workplaces is one of the causes of this low organisation rate. A 1983 survey by the Shinagawa Labour Administration Office showed that only about 10 per cent of establishments in this sector have been organised by trade unions.

Densanro (Council of Computer-Related Trade Unions) consists of 12 enterprise-wide unions and two area-wide unions which computer-related workers join as individuals, without regard to the companies they belong to. The latter type of union is unusual in Japan. The council has about 3,000 members and a full-time official. Although the council is small in terms of membership, it is very active in bargaining, research and policy formation. Recently, the area-wide union of Densanro in Tokyo has started a job placement service. Densanro has also submitted demands to the Japan Information Service Industry Association (JISA) concerning earnings by age groups, maximum overtime work and improvements in employment conditions of dispatched workers.

There is insufficient information to give a more detailed overview of labour-management relations in this sector. A few case studies, however, indicate that industrial relations in large and medium-sized firms in the sector are not unique in their procedural aspects.

Software development

Managers in the software business are trying to improve productivity by applying standardisation and computerisation techniques to software development projects. They are moving away from traditional programming, which has been characterised by the knowledge, skill and initiative of individual programmers, and are developing so-called "structured programming". Programmers who once did their work with pencils and coding sheets now operate terminals of specialised computers in which the programme for software development is loaded.

The goal in structured programming is to eliminate personal differences. Programmers structure programmes differently according to their preferences, with the same end result. This practice is said to be incompatible with an efficient division of labour. Structured programming was intended to allow all programmes with a large number of steps to be built from a small number of basic units.

The process of software development, especially large-scale programmes, is currently divided into clearly defined phases. In a typical case, it is composed of (1) system analysis, to analyse the tasks to be systematised in order to clarify objectives, effects, required human hours and costs and so on, resulting in a basic proposal; (2) basic system design, with a development plan agreed upon between users and developers; (3) design of system function, to determine the structure of software and input and output methods; (4) programming design to divide software into modules and to define how to connect them; (5) programming; (6) module testing; and (7) system testing to test the completed software. These phases may differ from one developer to the next. The results of these phases are documented in standardised forms. So far, computerisation in software development has been, on the whole, limited to programming and testing phases.

Usually system engineers are responsible for phases 1, 2, 3 and 7, while programmers are responsible for phases 4, 5 and 6. But sometimes the jobs of system engineers are distributed to system analysts and system designers. In other cases, the senior programmers who are responsible for phase 4 might supervise coders responsible for phases 5 and 6. A hierarchy thus develops which creates occupational distinctions between workers and the potential for degrading of occupations.

In cases where application software is developed jointly by user companies and software houses, problems may develop. If the software house participating in a project is in a weak financial or technical position, its workers are likely to be assigned less skilled jobs, regardless of other job-related factors.

How the computerisation of software production could influence jobs and skills is suggested in the case of Softward Company A, which introduced two specialised computers for software development. This company formed a planning section in charge of developing a software-writing system which works on the operating systems of the two computers. The system developed by the section has functions for simplifying operations, collecting data on schedules and actual work done by individual programmers, testing programme modules and so on. As a result, human hours required for programming are reduced to half and the number of errors has decreased remarkably.

When software production is computerised, programmers need a narrower range of knowledge than before to perform their jobs. Progress on jobs assigned to individual workers can be monitored. In short, while their jobs are easier than before, programmers have less room to plan and do their work according to their own preferences.

Dispatched workers

An important characteristic of employment in this industry is the large number of persons working on a "dispatched" basis. This means that workers of computer manufacturing and data-processing companies are loaned to user or client companies. From a 1982 MITI sample survey, it was estimated that one-third of the operators, about 20 per cent of the keypunchers and programmers and approximately 10 per cent of the system engineers are dispatched workers. However, a 1983 survey by the Shinagawa Labour Administration Office reported that 19 per cent of system engineers, 26 per cent of programmers, 60 per cent of operators and 33 per cent of keypunchers employed by firms in this sector were working at the workplaces to which they were dispatched. A survey by the

Ministry of Labour in 1983 showed that in 65 per cent of the cases studied, workers were dispatched for periods of more than one year.

Dispatched workers encounter numerous personnel problems. Accordingly, in June 1985, the Law Governing Proper Management of the Employee Dispatching Business and Improvement of Working Conditions of Dispatched Workers ("the Employee Dispatching Business Law") was passed by the 102nd session of the DIET.[6] It went into effect on 1 July 1986. This law seeks to clarify the division of responsibility between companies dispatching workers and those utilising their services. Some of the interesting provisions of the law are as follows:

- A company which dispatches only its regular employees is required to submit a report to the Minister of Labour before doing so. The company which registers workers in advance and hires only those whose skills are needed is required to have the permission from the Minister of Labour before doing so.

- The scope of this activity is limited to work where specialised knowledge, techniques or experience is needed and special employment management is required. These conditions will be fixed by a government ordinance after consultation with the Central Employment Security Council.

- Before dispatching workers, the dispatching company has to negotiate a contract with the receiving company on certain stipulated subjects (the nature of the work, length of stay with the receiving company, work hours, etc.).

- The dispatching company has to secure stable employment and training opportunities for dispatched workers.

- The receiving company has to nominate a person to handle grievances raised by dispatched workers.

- The legal responsibilities relating to employment fall on the dispatching company except for matters pertaining to working conditions, such as working hours and safety and health, which are under the control of the receiving company.

Other changes in jobs, skills and working conditions

At the first stages of automation, some operators were involved in operating programmes, but computers directed them on what to do at each stage. In general, operators' jobs are now becoming simple and repetitive.

Other simple and repetitive jobs are those of keypunchers and data-entry workers who are mostly women. Voluminous data-entry work is likely to be contracted out, especially if it occurs on an occasional basis.

A case study by the National Federation of Electrical Machine Workers' Unions of two relatively large data-processing companies suggested that the demarcation between system engineers and programmers as well as between programmers and operators was not rigid and that workers were promoted according to seniority and ability. However, it was uncertain whether the practice of promoting operators to programmers was common. Keypunchers tended to remain in the same occupation.

An opinion poll of union members of two data-processing service companies in 1982 by the Japanese Federation of Electrical Machine Workers' Unions, reported (1) that the workers satisfied with their work tended to emphasise the opportunities given to carry out their ideas; (2) that more workers wanted to move to better companies or start their own businesses compared with workers in other industries; and (3) that fewer workers expressed positive commitment to their company than in other industries.

The major causes of dissatisfaction related to wage levels, holidays and leaves, monotonous work, limited opportunities for self-development, shortage of workers, hours of work and welfare facilities. Operators and keypunchers were less satisfied than the workers in other occupational categories because of the lack of opportunities for self-development. However, rather a substantial number of workers reported that their jobs suited them.

A serious problem for workers in this sector is the great amount of overtime work and frequent night work. Workers are occasionally obliged to engage in extraordinarily long overtime hours, and frequently in exhaustive night work. The survey by the Shinagawa Labour Administration Office reported that 3 per cent of the sampled dispatched workers worked more than 101 hours of overtime a month and 21 per cent of them worked 51 to 100 hours. The main reasons for frequent overtime are that (1) the periods allowed for software development are, by contract, too short, due to the competition among software houses; (2) the specifications of software to be developed are often changed at the request of users; (3) unexpected errors or delays may happen at later stages; (4) computers cannot be used for development projects during the usual office hours of the users; and (5) workers may wish to complete a unit of work in a day or by a definite date. Of course, the trade unions have tried to regulate overtime and night work. The target of Densanro is to limit overtime hours to 50 hours a month. However, some managers argue that the working hours of computer workers, especially those of programmers, differ from those of the clerical workers engaged in routine jobs because computer workers are professionals and work intermittently.

It is commonly believed that computer workers cannot continue their jobs beyond 35 years of age. One probable reason for this is the overtime hours and night work involved. Another more obscure assumption is that older workers could not keep up with the rapidly developing technology.

According to the survey by the Shinagawa Labour Administration Office, more than half of the establishments surveyed in this sector pay special monthly allowances to system engineers, and about one-third pay special allowances to skilled workers.

The survey by the Shinagawa Labour Administration Office reported that, of 329 workers, 69 per cent complained of "weakened eyesight", 44 per cent of poor digestion, 37 per cent of fatigue and 34 per cent of headache or stiff shoulders. Of the workers who reported impaired health, 7 per cent had consulted doctors. Densamo made it clear that the complaints about "weakened eyesight" increased with the hours of operating VDTs.

Apart from physiological problems, possible psychological and social problems are also pointed out by a few doctors and reporters. As an example, it was pointed out that system engineers experience extreme psychological tension at the initial stage of operation of newly developed, large-scale software.

Technological and organisational options

Substantive aspects. Whenever users wish to install a large unit of application software, they have to decide if they will buy a ready-made package, develop it themselves or contract out all or part of its development. Almost without exception, large firms which have general-purpose computers are troubled with backlogs of software development projects. There are options for these companies: to let user divisions develop their own systems; to promote office automation of each division using personal computers and other machines; to improve the productivity of development project staff; and to use data-processing companies for the development or operation of their computers to save their own human resources. Computer manufacturers and software houses have similar options.

The expansion of computerised systems does not necessarily mean that specialisation relating to such systems will be common to all firms in the future. A substantial number of programmes owned by user companies are rather simple and developed by the system engineers and programmers of user companies who are not too specialised. This probably applies to data-processing companies too. In addition, software packages for personal computers, which are a fast-growing market, are manufactured by small-sized software houses in which workers are not specialised. There, however, is a tendency towards centralised control in this sector. This can be observed in the standardisation of various aspects of software development and the computerisation of programming and testing. However, a few companies in this sector as well as some EDP divisions of other companies have tried to promote quality circles.

Procedural aspect. Generally, a team is organised to carry out a large project. In this sense, the work of the sector is based on group work. The dispatched workers of a software house may form a sub-group or join the combined team as individuals. The employees of several companies may also form a group depending on circumstances.

As part of the implementation process of its computerised systems, the management consulted trade unions on their plans. This type of consultation differs from the established practices between management and the union. At a later stage, ordinary workers could participate in the improvement of daily work procedures.

Future perspectives

Data-processing industries are expected to expand as information systems develop. Software was originally written by hand but its production is increasingly being automated and, in some aspects, it now resembles the production process in factories. This trend is likely to continue for some time. Later, computer-aided production (CAM) of software will eventually include the phases of analysis and design.

At present, the undesirable effects of computer-based technology seem to focus on certain jobs, especially on those of junior programmers, VDT operators and keypunch operators. There seems to be limited options to improve these jobs through job design. The protection of these workers from undesirable conditions should become the focus of social policy.

Conclusions

Computer and telecommunication technologies have been developing rapidly. While their rate of diffusion differs according to the sector and the size of firms, it is clear that they are changing work in offices and commercial establishments.

The introduction of new technology may lead to new tasks or jobs which require new knowledge and skills. Computerised networks may influence communication patterns. The changes may affect categories of workers to varying extents, diminishing the content of jobs in some cases and expanding them in others. So far, the distribution of power among organisational echelons in Japan has not changed extensively with the introduction of computerised networks. However, some firms and local governments have tried industrial engineering techniques. These techniques to rationalise office work have resulted in specialised repetitive jobs, mostly performed out by women workers.

In spite of general improvements in working conditions, workers in the data-processing industry and VDT operators are faced with long hours of work and new health problems. Psychological stress is becoming a social concern in relation to the advanced technology.

Notes

1. See T. Shimada: *Nikonteki OA to sono tenkai* [Japanese-style office automation and its developments] (Hakuto-shobo, 1984).

2. The actual names of enterprises will not be used in order to maintain the anonymity of the companies studied.

3. Domei was dissolved and Rengo (the Japanese Private Sector Trade Union Confederation) was formed in 1987. Zensen and Shogyo-Roren (JUC) are affiliated to Rengo. The council of chain stores employers' unions has close ties with Rengo.

4. There are 23 special wards in the metropolis of Tokyo, with status comparable to cities. The metropolis of Tokyo itself is a local government at the prefectural level. The population of special ward A is approximately 270,000. Its ward office employs about 2,800 local civil servants, including about 30 EDP staff.

5. See M. Kainuma: "Chihojichitai ni okeru OA-ka to chihojichi no kiki" [Office automation in local governments and the crisis of local self-government], in *Keizai*, March 1984.

6. Japan Institute of Labour: "Outline of government and ministerial ordinance for implementing the employee dispatching business law", in *Japan Labour Bulletin*, 1 July 1986, pp. 6-8.

6 Applications of new technology in the private service sector of the Federal Republic of Germany

M. BAETHGE AND H. OBERBECK

Preliminary remarks

The following report examines the application of new technology in selected areas of the private sector in the Federal Republic of Germany. The areas selected for discussion – trade, banking and insurance – are those in which research has been conducted in the past few years.

The conclusions are based on our own research, statistics available from the Federal Bureau of Statistics concerning gainful occupations and from the Federal Employment Bureau concerning employees subject to obligatory social insurance, statistical surveys by trade associations and other empirical studies.

Changes in the rationalisation of office work

During the past two or three decades there has been considerable expansion in the services sector – in trade, in credit institutions, in private insurance companies and in various government units. It has been assumed that this expansion would continue, since no significant technical or organisational changes in the sector were foreseen. The special nature of service work, oriented as it is toward human communication and co-operation, was seen to permit only limited use of machines and technology in the labour process.

It is obvious that a central assumption in this analysis – that there would be no significant technical or organisational changes – is no longer tenable. Today, electronic processing affects not only routine and subsidiary functions but also qualitatively more demanding and complex activities, the so-called "brainwork" and communication and co-operation activities that were previously untouched by technology.[1]

As a result of the expansion of electronic processing, rationalisation efforts have not only increased but they have also changed in character. With traditional technical forms of rationalisation, mechanical aids were introduced into a clearly defined work process, and rationalisation effects were measurable quantitatively. Now, the introduction of more comprehensive electronic data-processing (EDP) systems is changing administrative and business functions in more complex ways.

Electronic data-processing (EDP) systems

Up to the mid-1970s, EDP systems were usually introduced on a case-by-case basis in certain departments or work processes. They were primarily employed where large quantities of homogeneous data had to be recorded and used to carry out relatively simple calculations. EDP use was concentrated in offices where money transactions took place, accounts were kept and where bookkeeping processes predominated. For the corresponding administrative departments (bookkeeping, payment transactions, sales business, cash accounting, credit accounts, post office accounts, savings accounts, etc.), separate individual data banks were installed for the batch processing of appropriate data and information.

During this time, it was found that series of simple and frequently repeated work processes could more or less be completely replaced by EDP. Subsidiary office functions, until then performed manually, were handled electronically. A related development was the restructuring of word processing operations, at first independent of EDP, in the registration and archiving of records and documents as well as in postal sorting and dispatch. To cope with an increasing amount of data and the constantly rising cost of labour, microfilming, separate machines for sorting data, mail and vouchers were introduced and subsidiary office functions (e.g. data registration and word processing) of service departments in credit institutions and insurance, and purchasing functions in trade, were centralised.[2]

Integrated microelectronically based EDP systems which contain storage capacity for data, information and control programmes are quite different from older EDP systems. The central elements can be briefly outlined as follows:

- Integrated data banks have replaced separate files for individual functional areas. This facilitates the processing of transactions and

172

communication between individual departments in a firm and also between a firm and its business partners.

- Considerably expanded storage capacity and better access to data allowt improved dialogue between workplaces.
- In view of the storage capacity now available, programs can be developed to process and control electronically stored data and information from various places of business. EDP can now be used as a management information system. This means that increasingly more programmes are being used for the qualitative assessment of existing business activities as well as for planning future policies.

System rationalisation of office work

The development of microelectronically based data processing and communication techniques facilitates system rationalisation.[3] System rationalisation processes are characterised by the fact that with the use of microelectronically based data processing and communication techniques, the combination of data, the organisation of business procedures and the control of various functions can be carried out simultaneously. Working within a defined boundary is supplanted by the process of working with an entire system. The routine elements of processing, such as data collection, data sorting, data documentation and word processing, as well as accounting operations, have been changed radically.

Trade, banking, insurance and public administration activities are essentially aimed at forming market relationships. The uses of new technology and the motives for rationalisation in those areas cannot be determined one-dimensionally (as, for instance, in production, where the primary aim of internal strategies is cost reduction). The rationalisation of service activities and administrative tasks must take into account co-operation and exchange with business partners, customers and clients.

Technically speaking, there are no foolproof solutions and there is no predetermined essential sequence for improving business administrative functions. The complete automation of individual work stages and procedures is feasible and results in office staff being guided in all details of their work. However, complete automation is no longer necessarily regarded as practical, or desirable, according to firm managers and rationalisation experts.[4] In some cases complete automation can be counter-productive to business goals.

The numerous methods of using EDP systems have provided a stimulus for organisational rationalisation measures. The existing division of labour has been permanently altered by the existence of simultaneous access to data banks and the possibility of up-to-the-minute alterations in the data bank by different departments. The more complex and inclusive methods of using EDP lead to a new pattern wherein subsidiary employees do the collection of data, preliminary sorting of information, archiving, documentation and winding-up procedures, and experts process the aspects of procedures (negotiations, qualitative assessment of applications, etc.) which are relevant to decisions. Changes in the division of labour at the decision-making level in the specialist departments and between specialist departments and management are increasingly the subject of a firm's rationalisation activities. Initial processing procedures which were previously undertaken in different places within the firm are increasingly combined in one operation, thus changing the job hierarchy.[5]

Developments in the wholesale and retail trade

With almost 2 million employees in 1982, trade is the largest employer in the commercial and administrative service activities covered in the study. In spite of a steep rise in the annual volume of work, the number of workers in trade has risen relatively little during the last two decades. The enormous discrepancy between rates of increase in work volume and employment implies extensive rationalisation.

Rationalisation took place during the 1960s and 1970s in connection with the introduction and rapid expansion of self-service shops and consumer markets, whose share in the market rose from 6 per cent to 13 per cent in just eight years (from 1970 to 1978).[6] The increased competition expressed in this development has forced other retail enterprises to rationalise.

Trends in rationalisation

The main trends in rationalisation for the retail trade (with consequent effects on the wholesale trade) in the past decade are the following:[7]

- a decrease in customer service relating to, for example, advice, delivery and repairs, with a move towards self-service;
- the centralisation of purchase transactions using new data processing techniques;

174

- the increased use of check-outs using electronic data reading devices, with the aim of creating continuously updated stock information systems; and
- more flexible arrangements of working time and capacity-oriented employment planning, with an increased use of part-time workers.

Progress in EDP development in trade seems relatively modest in comparison with development in other branches of the economy. There have been almost no fully automated sales statistics systems and/or registration of stock. EDP is used to automate partly the calculation of sales and/or inventory; a central computer is used to process punched cards which are filled in by the different branches. The information, in the form of printed lists, is made available to the buyers and sales managers either periodically (usually monthly) or according to need. This has the disadvantage of not being up to date and of giving only a limited amount of information, since for the most part only turnover data according to the types of goods are given or, in the food trade, order lists with stock listed according to article and suppliers.

A greater degree of EDP-type integration of commodity trade functions (EDP as a management information system) is planned, but in most cases such systems are only in the experimental stage. The final stage would be a fully automated listing of inventory, sales statistics and possibly also order calculations with the aid of an integrated, automatic stock information system which registers the stock on hand when the goods are price-marked. By means of check-outs using automatic reading or other electronic devices, sales would be registered according to the type of article, and essential characteristics (price, size, colour, etc.) would be stored in the central computer which would compile the data and make it immediately accessible via a screen or print-outs.

The development of organisational and technical rationalisation lies in the expansion and improvement of information systems. Large department stores and chain stores have been slow to install these systems and to create central data banks for the following reasons: the extensive organisational preparation required, the difficulties of building up a programme with a limited number of EDP staff, the lack of a standardised European-article-numbering (EAN) system in the area of foodstuffs; and problems in getting employees to use the EDP system efficiently. There are fewer such problems in the medium-sized retail trade, and, consequently the use of EDP is more advanced there. Completed conversions to EDP have led to a better understanding of the problems of introducing new data-processing systems, and this will hasten further developments. In general, however, developments are expected to be gradual.

At present there is no way to measure the effects of the new EDP technology on savings in personnel for the whole sector.[8] Direct savings in personnel are found primarily in administrative and bookkeeping departments. They usually relate to functions such as pricing, data input, cash audits, sales and stock control, and accounting. In these areas, further reductions can be expected with the increased expansion of EDP technology in trade. However, administrative work in trade takes up a relatively small proportion of the personnel. A further reduction in personnel can be expected in the next few years, but it will not be large when compared with the total number of employees.

Greater effects in employment are likely to be expected from the growth of automatic commodity control systems. Automatic commodity control systems give up-to-the-minute information on customer flow and the performance of sales personnel. With improved information and long-term planning, a new distribution of personnel can be carried out which helps to reduce personnel costs. The consequence is an increase in part-time work, flexibility in working hours and a reduction in employment.

According to this study, an increasing number of commercial enterprises are planning to employ personnel according to demand. The consequences will be an increasing proportion of part-time workers with irregular working hours and a permanent staff which, in its turn, is polarised into a relatively small group of qualified heads of departments, such as market managers, buyers, and so on, and a larger group which is "multifunctional", that is performing sales as well as administrative and inventory tasks. The management of commercial firms sees the potential for additional savings in personnel in this area.

The possibilities of using the new technology as an instrument of information and control over the flow of goods and customers, the distribution of staff or the organisation of the work process are by no means exhausted. No increase in employment is anticipated but a further slight reduction is expected in all types and sizes of commercial firms.

Developments in credit institutions and insurance companies

The mid-1970s marked a major change in banking policies because of several factors: a stagnation in the expansion of the branch network, a temporary peak in the organisational restructuring (e.g. mergers) in banks, as well as a major increase in the introduction of EDP especially in handling payment transactions. In addition, there was a slight drop in the expansion of business volume.

During the 1970s and the beginning of the 1980s, insurance companies and building societies had the goal of processing all transactions by paper-free methods to minimise the costs of filing, archiving and transporting documents. Increasingly since the beginning of the eighties, dialogue workplaces have been installed, that is workstations which use a VDU for two-way communication with a computer system. Paper-free processing will probably be as common as "automatic correspondence" (the calling-up of stored texts) in the second half of the eighties in all departments of insurance and building societies.

It is less clear how far computer-aided or computer-controlled processing will be employed. In principle, it can be assumed that in insurance companies, there are hardly any procedures or cases which could not be either computer-aided or computer-controlled. Likewise, it can be assumed that after the introduction of integrated data banks, hardly any technical barriers will remain for the computerised processing of all transactions. At present, however, it cannot be estimated how soon the enterprises will close the gap between the "utopia of the technically possible and the reality of planning and automation".

The reason for the uncertainty is the new expansion strategy held by banks since the second half of the 1970s. Savings banks, in particular, have taken on a pioneering role for the entire banking field. In the latter half of the 1970s, they replaced the traditional departments (e.g. giro accounts, savings accounts, security accounts and credit accounts) with a market-oriented organisation. Since then the entire industry has followed suit.

Trends in rationalisation

In the banking and insurance industries, the following trends in rationalisation can be discerned:

- the increased centralisation and automation of subsidiary functions by market-oriented activities (e.g. customer service and advice and processing of transactions and claims);
- a tendency to process transactions without paperwork by installing and expanding EDP-stored account and balance data banks;
- the start of computer-aided processing of transactions through the introduction of automatic correspondence systems and EDP-controlled processing of individual cases;

- the integration of the administrative structure through the combining of traditionally separate functions (e.g. integration of customer service and transaction administration); and
- the establishment of management information systems for the control of business expansion strategies.

Organisational changes have affected the division of work between tellers and customer service personnel, who look after accounts, and specialist departments, such as those dealing with credit transactions, security investment, and foreign transactions. These specialist departments are being disbanded in favour of an integrated customer service. In particular, a series of partial functions from the wide spectrum of credit transactions are being delegated to the counters.

In a market-oriented organisation, there is a new definition of the content of tasks to be performed. Employees are required to offer the customer a whole range of banking, investment and credit services. To accomplish this, customer advice zones have been established in the entries of main banks and branches. These are separated from the so-called fast-service areas (cash counters, places for the distribution of forms and statements of account). Such organisational changes are accompanied by the expansion of EDP into a management information system, used to control business policy approaches. Thus, the financial services required by the customer are evaluated so that they can be used as a basis for developing future sales strategies.

Computer-aided and computer-controlled processing programmes for customer advice and the handling of credit applications are envisaged in the near future. At present, however, it is not evident to what extent the use of such processing programmes is relevant for banks and over what period of time such a project could be realised.

Estimates of the future use of EDP in the area of customer self-service are to be regarded fairly sceptically. These estimates are based on the introduction of video display terminals principally in trade associations, credit institutions and insurance companies. Credit institutions and insurance companies, where the largest number of workers are now employed, are generally regarded as having the potential for a major success through the use of EDP, especially in their work with private customers. The general opinion, though, as expressed within enterprises and trade associations, is that such a development will not take place in the near future because of the cost involved and the fear of losing the opportunity to approach customers personally. The present competitiveness within the credit industry itself, as well as between credit institutions and insurance companies, places additional emphasis on

178

personal customer contact. Unlike insurance companies, credit institutions still have the advantage of being able to approach customers in their own branches more or less regularly. It seems doubtful that this strategic competitive advantage will be given up readily, just to increase the possibility of self-service.

Employment trends in credit institutions

According to national income accounting statistics, the increase in the number of workers employed in credit institutions continued to increase at a relatively high rate until 1970. Employment growth then dropped considerably and even stopped between the years 1973 and 1975. Since 1975 annual employment growth has been relatively constant at an average rate of 2 to 3 per cent. However, the growth rate in the volume of business has consistently been noticeably higher than the growth of employment. Between 1975 and 1982, the business volume of all credit institutions (including overseas branches) in the Federal Republic of Germany had risen annually on an average of around 10 per cent.[9]

There have been considerable structural changes in employment in credit institutions. Three developments which have a direct bearing on rationalisation initiatives are the following:

- Employment is stagnating or falling in those areas of banking where payment transactions are processed or where relatively homogeneous services are offered.

- The employment figures of higher paid groups are increasing, while those of lower paid groups are clearly decreasing; at the same time, the number of staff who are not specifically qualified for a particular occupation is steadily dropping.

- The proportion of males in the banking industry is increasing.

Different tendencies in employment can be established for individual groups of institutions in banking. For building societies and clearing-houses, there was a drop in the number of employees after 1981. However, since 1983 the number of staff in clearing-houses has begun to rise again. In those areas of banking where large numbers of relatively homogeneous transactions have to be processed (e.g. building loan agreements and settlement of turnover of payment transactions), the demand for employees has been decreasing in spite of the increase in the volume of business. In view of the relatively uniform type of processing in this area, intensive use of EDP was made very early on. The increase in productivity in building societies, essentially due to technical and organisational rationalisation, is apparent in the number of transactions per employee. Transactions almost doubled in ten years from 607 per employee in 1972 to 1,092 in 1982.

In comparison with building societies and clearing houses, the number of employees in private banks, savings banks and co-operative banks has risen continuously, with the rate of increase within the co-operative banks being the highest since the end of the 1970s.

The pattern of *qualifications of employees* also shifted in the second half of the 1970s. The proportion of employees with training in business consultancy, organisation and data processing has risen significantly. At the same time, the proportion of office assistants and those in unspecified occupations has decreased. These trends reflect the reduced demand for subsidiary work (in the area of payment transactions) and the increase in demand for EDP and organisation specialists.

The change in qualifications also had effects on the wage structure. Since 1972, in the private banking sphere the middle wage groups have more or less remained constant and the upper wage groups have doubled. A similar trend has been found in savings banks.

A major reason for the rise in qualifications, as evidenced by the shift towards higher paid employees, lies in the increased efforts of banks to provide expert customer advice service and to expand credit transaction facilities. Above all, credit institutions have pushed for a wide range of services and the diversification of credit financing and investment possibilities.

The *situation of female employees* in credit institutions has tended to deteriorate since the second half of the 1970s. The proportion of women in the total number of employees has decreased in particular in institutions where rationalisation has already been widely introduced.

In the near future the following rationalisation strategies in banking will be especially relevant to employment:

- Examination of the profitability of the branch network.
- Further expansion of regional computer centres which supply regional independent enterprises (e.g. the Länder of the Federal Republic of Germany) with all EDP services. This would not only cut the cost of EDP installations and programme development and provide an appropriate expert staff for individual businesses, but would also advance standardisation tendencies in payment transactions.
- The increasing use of EDP in the areas of customer advice and complex credit transactions and in those areas where a relatively high growth in staff has been noted. Additional rationalisation effects will emerge when paper-free processing is introduced everywhere. Areas

of work which require the preparation of material and information (compilation, calculations, archiving, organisation of return references) will become increasingly automated. Credit experts and customer consultants will have to deal with an increasing volume of work, which means that even with an increase in business, only a very limited increase in the number of employees can be expected.

- With the installation of integrated data banks in most of the credit institutions (by the end of the 1980s), extensive EDP programmes for cost analysis will come into use, leading to a more efficient use of staff. For example, this will recur in technically advanced institutions where customer consultants are employed and where lucrative business appears possible, while less profitable business areas are pushed into the self-service zones.

All these factors lead to the conclusion that credit institutions will need few if any additional personnel. If the economic development of the past years continues, credit institutions will in the medium term more or less hold their present level of employment. However, even with a slight increase (1 to 2 per cent), the idea that this employment-intensive area of the economy will be able to compensate for negative employment trends in other areas of the economy must be abandoned.

Employment trends in private insurance companies

Since 1975, employment in private insurance companies has stagnated, whereas the volume of work has risen. In office work, and particularly in policy administration,[10] new technologies have been introduced extensively and have led to an increase in productivity.

The decrease in the proportion of ordinary clerks, lower-level managers and secretaries in insurance companies underlines the close connection between rationalisation and employment. In the medium term, a continuation of the trend in employment in the private insurance companies can be expected. According to experts, savings of up to 10 per cent of the employment figure for 1982 can still be expected, even with continued business expansion. Additional increases in productivity will still be possible with the increasing integration of policy administration. Further decreases in lower-level, and probably also middle-level management (subsection heads), will occur. Expansion of paper-free processing, automatic correspondence and word processing will also reduce the demand for secretaries and office assistants. Computer-controlled processing or partial automation of frequent customer inquiries and modifications will lead to fewer routine tasks for qualified skilled workers and permit an increase in the amount of business handled by each employee. The insurance business will, in other words, continue to expand without needing additional staff, and even savings in employment seem possible to a certain extent.

Changes in job requirements: Simultaneous downgrading and upgraging of specialist qualifications

With the expansion of information and communication technologies to more complex activities, the nature of job qualifications has changed radically, and a new profile of behaviour is appearing. It is no longer adequate simply to ask the functional question: "What must a person be able to do to carry out his or her work?" It has become critical to look also towards the long-term competency which an employee must develop.

Jobs which involve interpreting situations, co-operating with others and evaluating information strategically are always more difficult to define than those where the work is highly segmented and unambiguous. For such jobs with "brainwork", it is difficult to write a precise job description because of the openness of the activities and the uncertainties or ambiguities necessarily present.

An upgrading of specialist qualifications is seen in certain areas, while dequalification tendencies are appearing in other areas. This development results from the increasing separation of internal administrative functions from market-linked functional areas, and from the computerisation of internal processing, checking and documentation tasks (such as the administration of insurance policies and the regulation of payment transactions). The introduction of EDP is changing the work of various skilled workers. Specifically, correspondence, checking and calculation processes have been transferred to the EDP system. The relatively few remaining skilled workers are mainly concerned with input activities, transmitting machine-produced analyses and passing on non-computerisable special cases. They have no contacts with customers and the work has no meaningful content.

For all the skilled workers involved, work now offers little stimulation to learn and is no longer regarded as being interesting or providing opportunities to retain or further develop their own qualifications. Instead, work is perceived and organised completely with the goal of reducing requirements, so that even the remaining challenging activities are detached and passed on to whoever can deal with them fastest. The new work situation in the long term leads to the indifference of employees,

182

which has negative implications for the future employment of skilled workers.

On the other hand, the new work pattern of administrative employees does not necessarily mean the complete loss of special skills. There is another line of development which is leading to the *upgrading* of qualifications. It provides increased opportunities to use professional knowledge and communications skills. The specialists involved are usually those dealing with the organisation of market processes (e.g. buyers, sellers and customer advisers in credit institutions, and experts and claims adjusters in insurance firms). The alterations in their work are usually the indirect effects of the introduction of new technologies, with the major emphasis being on changes in business policies following system rationalisation.

The following changes in the work of qualified specialists can be seen:

- The work content is increased, by an increase in the volume of independent decisions (e.g. by loan and credit experts), by widening the spectrum of tasks or by concentrating on complicated cases; usually there is a combination of several of these factors.

- There is nearly total computerisation of simple sequences, such as calculation, registration and checking processes in the handling of work. This facilitates concentration on more complicated cases and, usually, a compression of the time for making decisions.

- Different forms of electronic aid or control of work activity emerge (in the form of lists available regularly or upon request, direct access to stored information by means of the display screen, display-communicated control programmes for carrying out tasks), with the consequence of faster access to decision-relevant information and an equivalent pressure for faster processing of information.

- A compression of system-supplied communication or co-operation occurs (e.g. through the use of common data banks).

- There is an increase everywhere in the "transparency" of the work process and in the control of individual ways of working.

Though far-reaching, these changes are usually not recognised as structurally significant, because they are taking place slowly and in separate stages. They will, however, in various combinations, determine the future work of skilled workers in credit institutions, in insurance companies and in some areas of trade.

In order to operate successfully and to be promoted within the new structure of commercial administrative work, a professional style of behaviour is necessary which no longer has much to do with traditional "office tranquillity". It is characterised by less time to make decisions and by a more aggressive communication style with customers and/or suppliers. Mastering this new style depends upon being conversant in the area of work, having the flexibility to deal with changing situations, having the analytical ability to interpret information, and possessing communication skills. In the past, an employee's actions were supposed to be more careful and reserved, whereas now there is increased emphasis on aggressiveness and the willingness to take risks.

In contrast to the assumption that people could lose their control over production systems through the use of new technology, a clear upgrading of work skills and an increase in market-directed communication is occurring. The introduction of information processing and communication technologies has, as a side-effect, a more intensive use of human work potential and increased communication in the non-computerised part of business processes (which for the time being is still quite a considerable part).

Skilled activities in the work process can be described as complex procedures of information processing which are carried out for specific purposes. The degree of complexity and the qualifications necessary for their execution depend upon their content and upon the media available to process them. When the spectrum of tasks widens, or the frequency of decision-making increases, there is at the same time an increased need for professional knowledge and for conceptual and anticipatory thinking.

In electronic information processing the main challenge to the work style of qualified skilled workers arises from their use of data banks, which require them to select data from the large amount of information available and to decode or transform such data according to particular economic or social contexts. Both are complex intellectual achievements which often have to be carried out under relatively severe time pressure. Both require a high degree of professional knowledge, since it is only from such knowledge that a selective use of data banks can successfully be undertaken. Workers also require extensive professional experience to interpret the data.

We have focused on the pattern of qualifications of the most highly qualified types of work processing, since we assume that these will represent the main core of staffing in the future. The typical qualifications required for this group allow the dilemma of employees to be seen more clearly: their work situation does not contain anything which can produce or maintain the professional ability and intellectual activity demanded. This is especially true for credit experts and customer advisers in banks, for purchasers in central trade buying, for some of the claims adjusters in insurance firms, and for customer-oriented employees in local government. It applies to a lesser degree to employees in insurance firms and building societies who have to process less complex applications for services and to marketing managers and department heads in trade.

The spectrum of tasks for credit experts in building societies and for experts in the claims departments of insurance companies has expanded. Nevertheless, a sword of Damocles still hangs above the employee's head. Managers insist on a careful checking of claims in every individual case, even though such strict checking of individual cases may no longer be necessary or wise from the point of view of business policy. For marketing purposes, an unbureaucratic and accommodating handling of claims is preferred to the strict application of rules. The employee is thus caught between managers and salespersons. For credit and claims experts, the situation is even more critical, since organisation and personnel policy structures have, over the decades, sealed them off almost hermetically from those departments which deal with market analysis and the canvassing of new business.

In the case of department heads and marketing managers in trade, the diminution of responsibilities caused by the centralisation of purchasing and selling tasks need not necessarily go hand in hand with a major loss of professional qualifications. However, in the actual working environment, a change is taking place in the job description, with definite downgrading tendencies. The exclusion of department heads and marketing managers from supplier negotiations, and the issuing of standards on the kinds and pricing of items by a central office, are taking away from this group of employees not only their independence but also their motivation to gather more information on product quality and development. The expansion of electronically processed information (e.g. sales lists) available to them does demand more analytical work than before, but does not compensate for the loss of qualifications suffered, since this information does not allow much latitude for decisions.

Weakening of the position of employees

The main effect of the current technical and organisational changes on the work of employees appears to be a new structuring of skill requirements, not mass deskilling. In no way does this mean that we are announcing a new golden age for employees. Even where there is an increase in qualification requirements, with the introduction of the new technologies the position in the firm of the individual employee has been irreparably weakened. This is not solely due to new technologies, since there have also been changes in the labour market. But with the increased use of new technologies, the hierarchical relationships within firms change fundamentally at the expense of the employees.

We are not talking here of the major decisions or policies of the enterprise, but the basic day to day operations. We are talking about the distribution of opportunities either to fulfill the demands made by the enterprises in everyday working life or alternatively to escape from them, at least partially and temporarily. In the past, employees with specific expert knowledge or specific skills could hold back information from others or hinder its transfer. Until now, the activities of numerous mid-level employees and the special privileges and bonuses for employees within the firm (higher salary, better protection against dismissal, and so on) could be traced back basically to this characteristic of their work, with its limited visibility and controllability.

It is precisely this quality of their activity which is changed by microelectronic data processing. Even with increased integration and complexity of work, it is possible for management to make the smallest detail of the performance of activities visible and controllable. The genuinely epoch-making change in control lies in the fact that by means of the new EDP technology, not only the *results* of the work but above all its *course* can be monitored almost totally in its individual stages. This comprehensive possibility of control by itself means a structural weakening of the position of the individual employee within the firm.

In addition, this is occurring in firms during a time when there is available on the labour market a great supply of well-qualified applicants who all have advanced education or college training and often also have qualified professional training. Since this situation will not change in the foreseeable future, employees within the firm are under a double burden. How they will deal with it in their professional and social behaviour – whether by determined collective attempts to retain ground which is in danger of being irretrievably lost or by individual strategies in the form of increased continued educational activities and heightened competition and accommodation – cannot be forecast with certainty.

Notes

1 An overview of the connection between office rationalisation and its effects on employment is contained in P. Wenningmann and H. Oberbeck: *Die Bedeutung neuer Informations – und Datenverarbeitungstechnologie für Qualifikation und Berufsbildung kaufmännischer Angestellter aus der Sicht der Tarifparteien* (Göttingen, Ms. 1983).

2 F. Weltz, U. Jacobi, V. Lullies, and W. Becker: *Nenschengerechte Arbeitsgestaltung in der Textverarbeitung, Forschungsbericht Humanisierung des Arbeitslebens* (Munich, Federal German Ministry for Research and Technology, 1979).

3   M. Baethge and H. Oberbeck: *Zukunft der Angestellten (Future of the white-collar employee)*, (Frankfurt/New York, 1985). The translation "system rationalisation" used in the text does not adequately represent the content of the concept *systemische Rationalisierung*; the same applies to the term "systemic rationalisation".

4   Cf. the investigations by R. Koch: *Datenverarbeitung in der Industrie verwaltung*, No. 68 in the Series *Berichte zur beruflichen Bildung Beft* (Berlin/Bonn, Bundesinstitut für berufliche Bildung (BIBB), 1984); and also U Grünewald: *Elektronische Datenverarbeitung im Bankge werbe*, Heft 69, *Berichte zur beruflichen Bildung* (Berlin/Bonn, BIBB, 1984).

5   Rationalisation measures promoted by EDP control programmes are supported by modern marketing concepts, which aim at the principle of having customers or clients looked after by one person or having procedures processed by one expert. See M. Baethge and H. Oberbeck, op. cit.

6   ibid.

7   See E. Baker: "Einzelhandel 1990", in *Hauptgemeinschaft des Deutschen Einzelhandels*, (Cologne, 1980).

8   For a discussion on the methodological problems of available statistics and survey methods, and information on rationalisation in firms, see M. Baethge and H. Oberbeck: "Dienstleistungssektor als Auffangnetz?", in *Soziale Welt*, 1985, Issue 2, pp. 226 ff.

9   Quantitative figures for the business volume of credit institutes do not reflect the whole spectrum of banking, so that these data are not to be used uncritically as an indicator to describe changes in volumes of activity. (Cf. Deutsche Bundesbank: Monatsberichte 4/1971, p. 32, and Monatsberiche 3/1961, p. 31).

10   See, for example, "Rationalisierung in der Versicherungswirtschaft – Die Position der Arbeitgeber", special reprint from *Versicherungsivirtschaft*, No. 12, of 15 June 1982.

7 New technologies in administrative offices in Finland

L. RANTALAIHO

Introduction

There is currently a considerable demand for research on the impact of new technology on employment, work content, qualification requirements, the competitive capacities of organisations and efficiency. There seems to be an unconscious assumption that technological and social changes are beyond the control of people. But, of course, new technology is introduced and work is organised as the result of human decision-making.

Technology is planned, marketed, adopted and applied by people, and questions on technology should concern the people who control it and the objectives which they seek to attain. Likewise, it is important to study how people react in conditions of change, what strategies they adopt and how they integrate what is new and changing into their own activities.

To understand the actions of people, it is first necessary to understand the constraints involved in making technological choices. Case studies and surveys can then provide insight into the processes that take place. The present report on new technologies in administrative offices was prepared with that approach in mind. It was based on our project on office automation and women's work.

Our project, "Office Automation and Women's Work", consisted of two phases. The first phase resulted in an overall picture of the social conditions and consequences of office automation in Finland. Interviews were conducted with representatives of system suppliers, representatives of a broad range of mostly private user organisations, direct users of systems, consultants in the field, managing directors of firms which supply and hire out office workers, as well as several office workers themselves. The second phase consisted of case studies of the process of change when office automation was introduced in several government offices. The project, which took place between 1982 and 1985, was financed by the Research Council for the Social Sciences of the Finnish Academy. The research team consisted of L. Rantalaiho as leader, P. Korvajarvi as assistant and several graduate students.

Characteristics of the office sector

Growth in office work

Since the Second World War, Finland has experienced rapid and major changes in its industrial and occupational structures. Wage employment has become dominant in the formerly agricultural society of private farming. A second major phenomenon is the significant growth of the tertiary or service sector where most of the workers are women. The provision of welfare facilities and services has provided opportunities for women to obtain jobs in health care, education and social services.

Administrative and office work has increased rapidly everywhere in the society. This can be explained in part by the expansion of government agencies which went hand in hand with the creation of welfare services and social security systems. In the private sector, a similar expansion of administrative and office work took place with the increasing internationalisation of trade and finance. There has been a great relative increase in "information" work: work which, according to the classification of the Organisation for Economic Co-operation and Development (OECD), produces, processes, distributes and stores information.[1]

Characteristics of the labour force

Clerical and office occupations are strongly dominated by women. Of the main categories of clerical work in Finland in 1980, 95.8 per cent of the secretaries and typists were women; 76.0 per cent of the EDP operators and 84.8 per cent of those doing "other clerical work" were women.[2]

In administrative and clerical occupations, 60 per cent of the men are in managerial positions, both in the public and private sector, while only 4 per cent of the women are in managerial positions.[3] Generally, women are found in the lower positions in the hierarchy: fewer than 30 per cent of persons having supervisory duties were women, while over 90 per cent of clerical workers in routine work were women.

The rapid growth of administrative and office work between 1950 and 1970 exceeded the capability of the educational system to meet the educational needs of workers. Employers had to be satisfied with persons lacking specialised education for clerical jobs. The most typical educational background came to be graduation from "middle school" (nine years of general education). Women without vocational or professional training sought clerical work, while men in the same situation turned to industrial work. Today, most of the younger generation have acquired vocational training in the clerical occupations.[4]

The usual solution to the problem in education was to differentiate subsidiary tasks from other administrative functions and to create jobs simple enough not to require specialised training. At the same time, the rapid growth of agencies resulted in a hierarchical division of labour which differentiated between positions for men and those for women.

Women are often to be found in lower organisational positions, handling different routines. However, the size of organisations in Finland is not very large. Large Taylorised offices are not the rule. Even though the work is routine, it may be varied and relatively independent. In small – often local – organisations, office work need not be very compartmentalised at all. In larger organisations, clerical workers form a group whose work may differ according to autonomy, authority and work content. While office workers are women and the managers men, there is a middle group of staff specialists which may include men or women, depending on the branch in question.

For most office workers there is a definite career ceiling. In the public sector this is even reinforced by official regulations concerning the qualifications required. To move from office work to a staff or managerial position is not possible without certain educational certificates. In the private sector, the mechanisms are informal, but for the majority of office workers, just as rigid.

The great majority of women working in offices are married and have children. Many have interrupted their work career for a short time to take maternity leave or because of difficulties in finding day care for their children. Normally, however, they return to paid employment.[5]

Most office work is full-time. The frequency of full-time jobs differentiates Finland from other Nordic countries, where part-time work is quite common for women. According to a survey made in 1982, the proportion of part-time workers in Finland was 12 per cent in banking and insurance, 7 per cent in public administration, and 3 per cent in office work in manufacturing.[6] In most countries, part-time work is the way women enter working life. This is not so in Finland, where the participation of women in full-time, paid employment has traditionally been high – at present, 48 per cent of the labour force.[7] Part-time work is only a new development.

Office workers are relatively highly unionised. The great majority of their unions are affiliated to the central union, the Finnish Confederation of Salaried Employees (CSEF), which covers both private and public sector unions. The percentage of unionisation is estimated to vary between 80 and 95 per cent of all office workers. The unions of health care personnel with their almost total unionisation raise the average, but the clerical unions, too, are highly organised with 80 to 90 per cent of the potential membership. The large clerical unions are the Municipal Employees Union, the Finnish Federation of Industrial Employees (FFIE), and the Federation of Bank Employees (FBE).

Normally, collective bargaining in Finland is quite centralised. After signing the central frame agreement, separate unions sign their own agreements with employers' organisations – private, state and municipal. In larger organisations, clerical unions have their own (usually female) shop stewards. During the last ten years both the FFIE and the FBE have organised successful militant wage actions. There are also more timid new unions, such as the academically oriented Secretaries Association, which is developing from an alumnae association to a trade union with bargaining functions.

New technology in offices

Computerisation of offices has undergone two stages, a period of centralised computing and a period of integrated and decentralised information technology.

The first period started at the end of the 1950s. Banks and insurance offices were the first to adopt computers. Social security systems in the public sector were not far behind. The use of computers also spread rapidly in wholesale trade and industrial offices.

Computers were used in financial, economic and administrative routines like bookkeeping, invoicing, budgeting and payroll accounting. Computer functions were centralised in special departments, with specially qualified persons to plan and administer them, but also with a strictly hierarchical division of labour and highly differentiated routines. Information processing took place in batch runs, separate from the production of the information in time and place and requiring a large amount of manual preparation.

192

The second period of integrated, decentralised information technology has resulted from improvements in the cost, size and efficiency of terminals, text-processing systems and personal computers which have permitted their acquisition even by small organisations. At the same time, large companies are reorganising their former computer departments. The decisive organisational potential of the new information technology lies in its capability of handling real-time information, and its flexibility. This has led to decentralisation in information processing, and information technology has become a part of everyday clerical and administrative work.

The new decentralised information technology, however, has not completely replaced the older one. A 1982 survey of manufacturing enterprises indicated that there were no exclusively batch-processing or real-time system environments. Batch processing was found in 70 per cent of the organisations, while real-time terminal systems existed in 61 per cent.[8] The movement from batch-processing systems toward real-time systems was characteristic everywhere. Personal computers were rapidly becoming more common and, by 1982, they were used in 42 per cent of both large and small enterprises. Text-processing systems were used in 31 per cent, but larger integrated office automation systems existed in only 10 per cent of the enterprises. Both text-processing systems and larger integrated office automation systems were more common in the larger enterprises.[9] From the public sector some absolute numbers are available. During 1982 the number of text-processing systems in government administration was estimated to be 200. At the beginning of 1984, around 1,000 computers and 6,500 terminals were in use in government administration (personal computers not included). The absolute numbers are naturally misleading, since all sources estimate the yearly increase to be very rapid – for example, text-processing systems should double every year.[10] Government plans for office automation systems in public administration would result in two-thirds of the clerical and administrative employees of the government using new information technology in their work by the end of the 1980s. In municipal administration, the number of terminals increased by 57 per cent during 1980; by 1985 this number was expected to have more than doubled.[11]

Government and union policy on new technology

At the end of the 1970s the micro-electronic revolution was the talk of the day. International competition had sharpened, and micro-electronics was expected to create new opportunities for the countries which could react quickly. The Finnish Government organised its own Technology Committee to evaluate the technological developments and to create action programmes.[12] By 1980, the basic guide-lines of the government's technology policy were ready: a strong emphasis on the promotion of new technology to guarantee national competitiveness. Besides the political programmes, a network for the cultural and ideological promotion of new technology was created, and has been active these past years. Conferences, seminars and publications reinforce the consensus for "moving Finland to the era of the information society". A visible part of the publicity is the marketing of information technology and office automation systems. The intensive advertising creates a background for people to see the new technology as being "as inevitable as tomorrow".

Trade unions in Finland, unlike those in other Nordic countries, have not been very active in technology policy on behalf of their membership. With one notable exception in the early 1970s in the graphics industry, trade unions have not concluded special technology agreements. Technological change has not appeared as an independent question in collective bargaining. Branch agreements and records of negotiations contain occasional references to the anticipated consequences of technological change, such as security of employment, need for retraining, maintaining occupational categories, and so on. However, the question of new technology or technological changes in general is both conceptually and practically subordinated to other aspects. The dominant view sees technological change as part of a process of rationalisation. As such, technological changes are part of the employer's right to manage and control the work. This way of thinking has made it difficult for trade unions to adopt an active policy of their own. However, the trade union movement in Finland has traditionally supported technological change. In recent years, the ideological appeal is expressed in terms of modernity and national competitiveness.

New information technology has been discussed quite a lot among the white collar unions since the 1970s. The focus of discussion has been the threat of unemployment. Clerical unions are also especially interested in ergonomic problems and the development of work content. Several clerical unions have formulated their own programmes for ergonomic requirements in terminal work.[13] The Finnish Federation of Industrial Employees has published a review of technology agreements in other European countries and has pushed for an agreement for themselves. So far the resistance of employers' organisations has been too strong. However, in banking, trade unions have been able to achieve a common scenario for future technological and personnel developments.

The most controversial question in technology policy is the workers' right to participate in the planning and control of the processes of change. The Finnish Government, for example, set up a special committee of worker representatives, chaired by an official of the Ministry of Social and Health Affairs, to discuss and propose forms of worker participation in the introduction of new technology. When this committee delivered its report, each member – excluding the chairman – added an official disagreement to the "common" report, so that the major part of the text consists of expressions of disagreement.[14]

Employers in the private sector may take a rigid standpoint of "no participation rights" in official contexts, but in their own firms many employers adopt a modern management style of including their employees in project groups on technological change. In the public sector, new technology is handled as part of existing rationalisation agreements. There is a central agreement for municipal workers concerning procedures for organising the participation of employees in connection with automation.[15] Implementation of this agreement depends on local initiatives. In government administration, technological change is directed by the Ministry of Finance. Government decisions state that no one will be dismissed because of the introduction of new technology. Departments develop retraining and transfer plans in case of redundancies.[16] The collective agreement with government employees defines some participation possibilities for the personnel. Here again, the practical consequences are very much dependent on the degree of local activity.

Effects of information technology on clerical occupations

Changes in employment structures

Early forecasts on technological change predicted dramatic unemployment in offices. This has not taken place. Instead what is clear is that the growth in clerical occupations is tapering down.[17] Some of the specialised functions and jobs created during the early days of computers, dealing with preparatory routines for batch processing and data entry, have almost disappeared. Otherwise, not much information points to direct unemployment effects.

The demand is for highly educated technical specialists, computer system planners, software experts, managers and marketing experts. According to the Finnish Confederation of Technical Employee Organisations, industrial wage statistics showed a personnel growth during 1981 to 1983 of 19 per cent for upper-level white-collar employees and managers, 2 per cent for technical employees and 1.5 per cent for clerical employees. This indicates more opportunities for persons with college education, in technical or economic fields, and fewer for persons without college education or with non-technical education. Taking into account the sex segregation of occupations, this points to employment difficulties for women.

New information technology eliminates small parts of the tasks of several persons, and reductions of staff can only be achieved through rearrangement of the job content. Usually no one is dismissed, but internal transfers to other jobs may take place. Moreover, when employees leave – retire, take another job, or go on extended maternity leave – they are not replaced. A reliance on natural wastage predominates, both in the public and the private sectors. Entrance and re-entrance to the labour market is becoming more difficult, in particular for women.

Within organisations the introduction of new technology only seems to improve career advancement possibilities of office workers in a few isolated cases. Some possibilities for improving careers exist for those with a good educational background, but usually not in their own organisation. Instead, there have been cases where workers took jobs with the system supplier of their former organisations.

Some experts in information technology and marketing point to the possibilities of freeing information work from its bonds of time and place. This could give women a chance to do their office work at home, while fulfilling their responsibilities and obligations towards home and family. In Finland, this kind of remote work has not been planned or put into practice on any large scale. Office workers themselves and trade unions were unfavourably disposed to the idea. Some programming work has been done away from the main office of a software house, but not at employees' homes. Working with home terminals, however, is likely to become more common, especially with highly qualified experts and specialists who are full-time employees and with the self-employed who have their own small businesses or who want to earn extra income by working evenings and week-ends.

Part-time work as such does not directly increase as a consequence of new technology in the clerical occupations. None of the organisations interviewed had adopted part-time hours. Statistics show a slight increase in part-time work in the banking and insurance industries. This usually means that now and then some of the new employees are engaged on a part-time basis, while the old personnel remain in full-time jobs.

However, a new marginal labour force is emerging in the larger towns: temporary office workers hired by special service firms. In Finland this is a new development. This temporary labour force is not a consequence of new technology, but is an indication of a general economic trend toward the flexible use of labour. In this segment of the labour market, special qualifications and experience with new information technology are certainly in demand. For the firms using the services, it can even be a way of saving training costs. Employers can use women's problems, their paid work and their family responsibility, as well as their secondary position in working life, to get a flexible and mobile labour force. This means, however, that the solution to organisational needs is to use flexible labour instead of flexible ways of organising work.

Working with new information technology

While information technology has not led to drastic employment effects, its use has meant many changes in the way people do their jobs.

The Central Statistical Office of Finland conducted a comprehensive Working Conditions Survey at the end of 1984 with a sample (n = 4,502) of the economically active wage-earning population.[18] This survey included several questions about new information technology. Approximately, 17 per cent of the wage-earning population were using new information technology regularly in their work. Most used it only as a small part of their work, but it was a major part of their jobs for one-third of the respondents. Clerical workers were the biggest users by far.

The new technology is mostly used for retrieval or dialogue. Common methods of application include compiling statistics and making reports; maintaining registry files (of clients, patients, products, etc.); buying, selling and invoicing; research and planning; keeping stock records; customer service (account positions, reservations booking); text processing and bookkeeping.

The survey showed that 64 per cent of the users reported that they previously did the same kind of work manually. Even if the new information technology has changed the way they do their job, the job itself remains the same.

However, there were indications that characteristics of the job such as the requirements of the work, the level of responsibility, pressure of work and mental stress have increased, while physical stress and contact with colleagues have decreased. While this cannot be interpreted as degradation of work, it does point to important problems.

197

Most of the users are doing their former jobs with technically more developed tools. Their position is not upgraded in the organisation because of that, although there are other, informal processes at work.

The pressure of work has increased because the quantity of information to be processed has multiplied. Since the technology is there, much more than before should be accomplished and, certainly, at a much faster rate. Supervisors or managers often have an unrealistic picture of the limits of a system which they themselves do not use directly. Although in some cases it is true that users do find it easier to meet peak demands since many former routines have disappeared.

A survey of its members by the CSEF in 1984[19] showed that the greatest problem in the work environment was mental and social stress. The two most commonly mentioned problems in working conditions were "hectic pressure and rush", experienced by 36 per cent, and "too few personnel", experienced by 26 per cent. The most common improvement was "better lighting", cited by 11 per cent. The most frequent reasons given for both the improvements and the problems at the workplace were "technological change", "new technology" or "automation".

Problems in the introduction of information technology

The introduction of new information technology results from both internal and external pressures such as bottle-necks and back-logs in information processing, long-term objectives of cost reductions and the marketing efforts of system suppliers. Information technology is mainly introduced for economic reasons. In large organisations this includes consideration of savings in labour costs and the possible profitability of new kinds of services, while in small- and medium-sized organisations the economics of information technology are viewed more as a bargain with the system suppliers (how much support and maintenance can be included, is the system open for development later on, will it fit together with the existing technology, etc.). Such decisions are the domain of managers, and where special expertise is needed, the services of consultants are contracted. As a rule, this planning and decision-making process takes place without consultation with office workers. Where planning is delegated to special project groups, which is often the case in large organisations, office workers are mostly "represented" by their department superiors. Office workers have no say in the matter of "representation".

The object of planning as far as office work is concerned is to get a quantitative picture and a formalised model of the information processing which takes place in the organisation. Typical questions include where office work is done, how different sub-routines are combined, what the information flows are, and what needs to be archived. Copy typing is one of the most commonly analysed functions.

In the introduction of new technology, great emphasis is put on warding off the resistance of users to change; even special attitude training is arranged. It is desirable that the user, commonly a woman, should be motivated and interested in taking up new technology as a tool, but basically it is not expected that she should be interested in participating in, or actively making suggestions for, the planning.

On the contrary, too much interest and a desire to participate in making the rules are often interpreted as resistance to change. The user should be enthusiastic, but active only in those matters on which an opinion is asked. The user must thus be active within the limits set by others, above all by the management and the experts, and within the boundaries of their operational ideology. Users usually have no chance of moulding the structure of participation in planning the introduction of new information technology.

The introduction of new information technology could mean a planned change of work organisation in administrative and clerical work. Instead, what mostly takes place is a process of allocation of equipment within the existing organisation of work. The consequences are often manifested at the level of the social community of the workplace, in group relations and social tensions. Another point is that the use of information systems often requires a lot of ad-hoc inventiveness from office workers who, through their knowledge of the organisational environment, fill the inevitable gaps and act as interpreters between the formal categories of data processing and the real life surprises that the machines cannot deal with.

In the field of new technology, there also seems to be a definite place for technological determinism: marketing and advertising promise freedom from boring tasks as soon as the hardware is moved into the office. The cultural values of progress and modernity give a positive glow to all changes. The promises emphasise ease of use: anybody can perform better with these shining tools. The concrete work process in offices, however, is not just button-pushing. Therefore, the problems of discrepancy between the actual requirements of the information system and the weakness of the marketing promises become pronounced.

The nature of office work

The common conception of office work is that it is a conglomerate of routines which can easily be replaced by an information system in the computer. Our observations about the reality of office work aroused suspicions as to the validity of that view. Eleanor Wynn also comes to a different conclusion in her study concerning the content of office work.[20] She describes office work as a daily problem-solving activity which cannot even be described accurately enough to be entirely translated into the language of programmes and information systems.

Wynn discovered that ordinary office workers were constantly describing and explaining situations to each other. They often told each other the background of matters or the connections between them, especially when solving problems. At the same time they developed a common understanding of their work and its objectives. This social interaction of office workers can be called a form of production in which common interpretations and explanations for matters are constantly and repeatedly created, restructured and reinforced.

Office work in fact requires that its performers should have a common frame of interpretation to which the matters conveyed to others can be related, both inside and outside the office. Information passed on in the office is thus both the product of activity and its instrument. A certain social and cultural world, traditions of the work community, customs and habits are shared in daily work, in interactions between people, and are thus made common property. Various kinds of incidents, on the basis of which things are given their meanings, interpretations and backgrounds, are related to them.

The essential purpose of office work is to produce, distribute, convey, rearrange, apply and interpret information of various kinds. The content is by no means unambiguous and visible, nor can the work done in the office be reduced to a visible new product, as in material production. On the contrary, it is a question of maintaining the past in order to guarantee continuity in the work group and in the whole work organisation. The continuous production and maintenance of common frameworks of interpretation is an activity of which even office workers themselves are unconscious to a great extent.

The "community" produced in office work, both by common frameworks of interpretation and by common usages, is generated and kept up without the workers themselves knowing it. In this process, things which are obvious and predictable are mixed with things which are obscure, emotional and unexpected. Yet the quality and usefulness of the information which is passed on in the office is dependent on these commonly maintained and generated assumptions and frameworks of interpretation.

How is this view of office work to be reconciled with the prevalent understanding of offices as "information factories"? Is clerical work not broken up more and more into simple routines, standardised and formalised?

In large offices with functional divisions of labour – for instance large insurance offices, post offices, main offices of wholesale trades, etc. – work is strictly divided between departments and every single worker performs his or her specific partial task from morning to evening.[21] These are the visible offices, the prototypes of "proletarianisation" of clerical work which are discussed in numerous sociological treatises.[22] They represent the "modern" office, a model towards which all other offices are expected inevitably to evolve. The rest of them are just "vestiges", according to this theory. This view also leads to a prediction of large unemployment and degradation of work as a consequence of technological change.

But the "vestiges" stubbornly resist the predicted development. We maintain that this is so because they actually have another kind of work organisation which is more effective. The tasks that office workers perform are variable and not easily standardised; many of them are routine, but are often performed in unpredictable combinations and contexts. There is limited functional division of labour. The important thing is that these offices are very common. You find them both in the public and in the private sector. With the small average size of organisations found in Finland, these offices make up the majority of clerical workplaces. During the period of growth it may have seemed that all offices would develop toward the "Taylorised model", but at the present time the "traditional" office emerges as the viable model.

But there is inside these traditional offices another kind of invisible mechanism at work: patriarchal relations and gender division of labour. On the one hand, it is a question of power, on the other hand, of maintaining people's personal identity. A sex-segregated labour market with women in clerical occupations results for example in a difference in wages. But the consequences go deeper than that.

Training: Discrepancy between marketing promises and job requirements

Training is arranged on the basis of marketing promises. It provides superficial learning of isolated operations. Training usually does not exceed two days; it is provided by the system supplier as part of the package, often to one or two office workers, who are then supposed to instruct their fellow workers. The training does not cover any theoretical knowledge of the information system as a whole, which would make it possible for the user to consciously analyse the information system of the office in abstract terms. In addition, the software is often sold and bought in standard packages which do not allow much flexibility of use.

System suppliers must obviously operate on the basis of their marketing promises. User organisations for their part do not consider it profitable to invest in the training of women at the lower levels of the hierarchy. And since the new technology is expected to perform effectively, office workers are seldom given enough opportunities to practise and to familiarise themselves with all the possibilities of the new systems. As a result, the system's potential is never realised.[23]

The discrepancy between the training which is considered sufficient and given to the users and the actual requirements of the work is handled by thrusting the responsibility for mastering the information systems onto the users as individuals. Emphasis is put on the office worker's individual work orientation, positive attitude, enthusiasm, courage and initiative. The suppliers as well as the management in organisations regard the mastery of information systems as dependent on specific personal attitudes. A certain kind of work orientation, in other words, acts as a source of motivation for learning new practical skills. The user's individual motivation is the solution to adjusting the discrepancy between the training provided and the requirements of the job.

This affects the social community of office work. To be chosen as a user of the system and to work with expensive and modern technology is a kind of reward and recognition. A few "capable" users may rise up to the position of trainer of other workers. This is usually done unofficially and does not result in an increase in salary or redefinition of job content. Instead, it sometimes leads to social isolation of the worker in question.

However, in some cases, co-operation between users with similar problems has become stronger. A new information system has sometimes encouraged users, superiors and experts at higher levels of the hierarchy to co-operate with each other. This gives the users opportunities to extend their professional competence, to acquire an overall picture of the activities of the organisation, and to relate one's contribution or part of it to the overall work process.

Case studies

Background

The Ministry of Justice was in the process of developing its information system on the basis of new office technology and invited us to make a study of the consequences of the changes on women's job opportunities. Two central administrative offices and two smaller local courts were chosen. The Ministry gave authoritative support so that access for lengthy observation and interviewing was relatively free. Four case studies describe the introduction of the new information technology in these offices.

The two central administrative offices were both located in the capital. Each office had about 75 to 80 employees. One of them, (PA), was responsible for co-ordinating and managing the Finnish prison administration. Therefore, a great deal of the department's activities were involved with the legal and financial control of other institutions around the country. Outside contacts were mostly with organisations rather than with individual clients, so that there was not much client service in the ordinary sense.

The other central office (CA) was a special court of appeals of pension and insurance cases. Any citizen could appeal an insurance or pension decision. Most contacts were with individual clients, but the office also regularly contacted other special organisations and professional consultants.

The two local courts (LOC/H and LOC/T) were both situated in small towns in the region of the capital. Each serviced a population of about 75,000 and had a similar number and composition of civil and criminal cases and administrative legal functions, such as keeping registers of titles, mortgages and inheritance. All these matters require substantial services to individual clients, lawyers and banks.

The following table summarises the personnel structure in each organisation studied:

Office	Management positions	Intermediate positions	Office workers	Total
PA	1+4	44	35	84
CA	1+16	18	18+15+2	70
LOC/H	1+3	4+2	10+3	23
LOC/T	1+3	4+2	9+1	20

All permanent office workers in all the organisations studied were trade union members, but for most of them that was a formality.

All of these offices were under the central control of the Ministry of Justice. Their functions and organisational goals were defined by laws, statutes and instructions, and their economic and personnel policy decisions were tied to the budget of the Ministry's central offices. Especially in the court of appeals and the local courts, the law guided the daily operations in great detail. There existed an important link to the centralised administration which was not relevant to the research: the Ministry had its own large planning unit for the development of its information systems (ISU) which was geographically separate in a city in southern Finland. For all of these offices there were various degrees of dependency and outside control, and all had their gender-differentiated personnel structures.

At the beginning of the case studies, several information systems were being introduced or prepared for introduction in various offices under the Ministry of Justice. These included a register of legal precedents (already in use in the higher courts); local registers of real estate and en-cumbrances; systems of direct fining of minor offences; registers of applications for unarmed military service; registers of the recording and execution of court decrees, and so on. Many of these systems concerned information of importance to several different authorities, so that in many cases mailing of copies could be simplified with an electronic mail system. The ISU of the Ministry took care of planning common systems and also centralised the compilation of registers from accumulated local data. Larger departments had the option of planning their own unique internal systems. The systems and technology introduced in the offices studied included both computer-based larger information systems and "local" text-processing systems, or some combination of these. They concerned both the functioning of the offices as a whole, and also individual parts of their operations. (In talking about office technology or new information technology, the essential part referred to is not the hardware but the information systems).

Short visits were made to the offices to describe the research and its aims, discuss the practical arrangements of the studies and establish a contact person in each office. Shortly before the actual installation of computer systems and terminals, we presented a questionnaire about the expectations people had of the new systems. A second questionnaire was presented, after about a year of use of the systems, to examine what workers had experienced with the changes.

There were two periods of intensive observation and interviewing in the study, the first immediately before and during the introduction of the new technology, and the second after about half a year of its use. The observations covered the functioning of the entire organisation, social relationships and the organisation of work, but were most detailed in the case of office work. The interviews concentrated on office workers, but naturally included other groups as well. The themes of the interviews included planning and decision-making, the development of work organisation and the division of tasks in the offices. In the case of office workers, the interview also went rather deeply into work histories and orientations.

During the research process we had regular feedback meetings with the office workers. Questionnaire results, progress in the use of the information systems and any problems encountered were discussed. Several group interviews with office workers concentrated especially on the problems of their work.

We also interviewed several persons working in various positions in the ISU: managers, computer specialists responsible for the development of the information systems, office personnel who had the input tasks in the registers, and personnel with training and advisory functions during the period of introduction.

Planning

Planning of the new information systems had begun during the 1970s in the Ministry's planning unit (the ISU). Several larger departments of the Ministry of Justice had also prepared reports on their information flow and on possibilities for rationalisation. An ISU newsletter emphasised a democratic approach in the planning. For example, it stated that future users of the information systems should participate in the planning and that experts should have contacts with the people actually doing the work – the office workers and clerks – and not only with their superiors. Such was the content of public pronouncements, but frequently the reality was different.

The computer-based information system in each of the offices studied was part of a branch-wide development plan and was therefore tied to the ideology and organisation of the branch. The ties to the consultant organisation varied, but on the whole the larger departments with their own resources were more independent, while the smaller units relied more on outside specialists. Still, even in the smaller units, strategies could differ greatly depending on other ideological and organisational commitments (such as those to the trade union movement).

The government budget system also created constraints, which resulted both in timetable difficulties and, later on and in the case of ergonomic problems, in weaknesses of planning.

The planning in each of the offices studied proceeded separately from the everyday work process. Participation by workers was far from the ideal expressed in official public statements. The office workers were not expected to participate in planning and certainly were not given the possibility of participating effectively.

The office workers served as information sources about their work for the planning teams, but were not encouraged to decide what information would be relevant or important. The office workers in LOC/H were a partial exception to this rule. They had their own working group to discuss problems of work organisation and made suggestions about the system programme to the ISU experts.

The planning was rather abstract: general development, rationalisation and faster information flow were the objectives. Inside the offices, these objectives were taken as given. The practice of office work remained invisible, and plans dealt only with the formal flow of paper and the quantity of typed material. Choices and decisions about work organisation and social relations in the division of tasks between people were neglected, often because they were not even considered as possible problems, but sometimes also because the existing power structure was obstructive to changes. Some of the general features of the planning process were thus structural constraints, the formal computer-centred system plans and the exclusion of intended actual users from the planning process.

Expectations and experiences with new technology

The process of planning and waiting brought into the offices an awareness of changes to come. People discussed the new systems, expressed their doubts and hoped for the best, mostly on the basis of office gossip and hearsay. Beforehand employee attitudes were characterised by uncertainty and suspense on the one hand, but on the other hand, trust that the situation at their workplace would remain essentially the same.[24]

Shortly before the systems were introduced, the main problems mentioned by the future users were "lack of information" and "lack of possibilities to participate". Seven out of ten thought they did not have any part in the planning process. This varied according to organisational position, so that half of the managers, two out of three in intermediate positions and five out of six office workers felt they lacked opportunities to participate in planning the introduction of new technology.

A striking example of the lack of information was that at the time of the questionnaire (just a short time before introduction of the changes), 41 per cent of the respondents did not yet know whether they themselves would be using the new systems or not, and the level of uncertainty was even higher among office workers as a group. This meant that for an individual, his or her actual relationship to the new technology would only be determined when the hardware had arrived and the system was being introduced. Superiors, colleagues, internal communications and in-house training served as the main sources of information.

The responses to the question on qualification requirements for using the software and hardware of the new information systems to be introduced could be grouped under four categories: personal and motivational qualifications, traditional office work qualification, technical qualifications concerning computer-based systems and terminals, and general knowledge about computer science and systems design.

The differences between personnel groups were widest in the evaluation of traditional office qualifications. Those in management positions more often emphasised traditional office competence and gave less importance to specific technical qualifications and wider conceptual mastery of computer systems. More than half of the office workers, on the other hand, stressed precisely those aspects. The people in higher organisational positions systematically estimated the qualification requirements to be lower than the office workers themselves did. What was common to all personnel groups was that the personal and motivational qualifications headed the list.

Certainly the respondents also had other problems and doubts about office automation. To an open question about the expected negative consequences, the single most common answer was the threat of unemployment. Four out of ten office workers mentioned it. This was, however, a general social problem to the respondents, and very few actually had personal fears of losing their own jobs. They knew about the rationalisation plans of the government, but felt rather secure in their own organisations, since there were so far no explicit plans to reduce personnel. Still, when we consider all the most common negative consequences mentioned – threat of unemployment, impoverishment of work content, health problems and work stress during the transition period – four out of five such problems were experienced by women. Men were not as worried; four out of ten mentioned explicitly that there would be no negative consequences. Positive consequences were indeed expected by most of the respondents.

Characteristically, these positive expectations were rather vague, and mainly concerned some kind of overall improvement in work. It is easy to see the reflection of public ideologies of technological progress and the language of advertisements. Six out of ten respondents expected "less routine and more meaningful work".

The concrete expectations of improvement centred around better customer service with quicker information flow and fewer mistakes, which seemed especially important for the courts. When asked specifically to mention consequences for their own organisation as a whole, about half mentioned improved efficiency and flexibility – the vocabulary of the general advertising language.

The only negative consequences mentioned by superiors were the organisational problems of the introduction and transition period. Expectations of improvement in work content did not appear at all in this context, and relatively few also mentioned the better customer service. Office workers found it hard to mention anything besides "efficiency" and vague doubts about social consequences.

Structured questions about the aspects of one's own work which would improve, worsen or remain as before, produced a coherent picture of expectations. First, the status quo was expected to prevail in the case of one's salary (96 per cent), organisational position (94 per cent), appreciation of one's work (90 per cent) and even security of employment (87 per cent – here the people who had doubts were office workers).

Secondly, most respondents expected the new technology to increase the quality of service that clients would receive (78 per cent), the functional flexibility of their department (71 per cent) and even the efficiency of work (62 per cent).

Thirdly, there were some interesting differences in attitudes concerning organisational position. For example, superiors were mostly optimistic while office workers were generally pessimistic with regard to working conditions, work content, and solidarity and group atmosphere at the workplace. There was, however, one aspect where office workers had high hopes: they expected to be able to improve their qualifications (see figure 1).

The pattern of expectations reflects the process of planning and introduction. Work organisation with its attendant consequences would remain as it had been, the hierarchical rock of stability. Technological change would just give a boost to organisational functioning. Superiors had an altogether rosy view of the future in their department, while office workers tried to cope with doubts, hoping for a chance to improve their qualifications.

After the new information systems had been in use for about one year, we studied the situation again. The period of transition was over, and the system had mostly settled down to a routine.

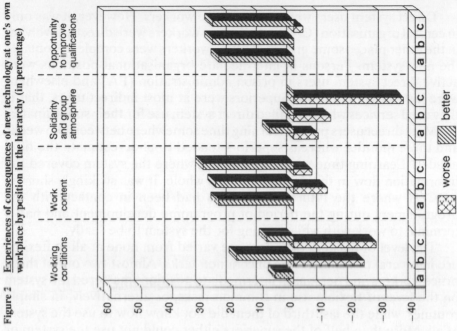

Figure 1 Expected consequences of new technology at one's own workplace by position in the hierarchy (in percentage)

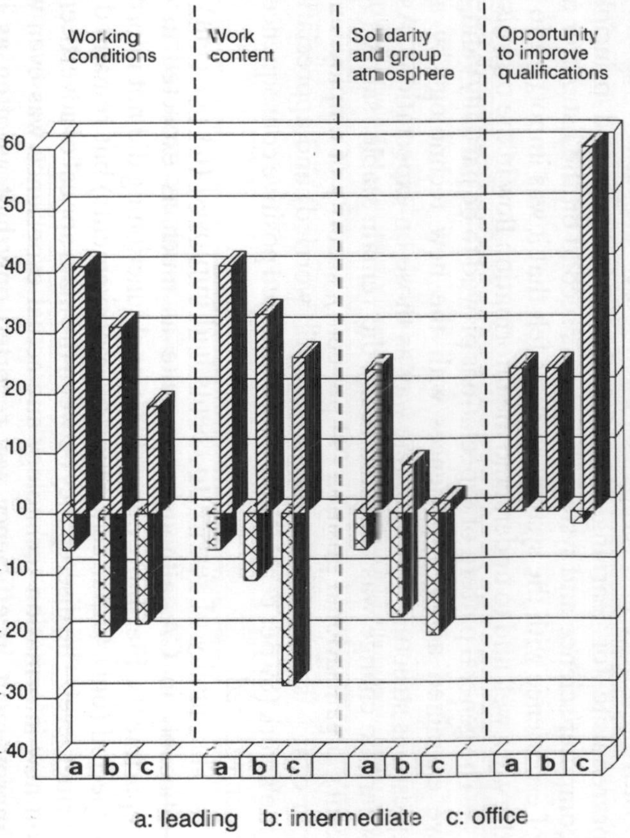

Figure 2 Experiences of consequences of new technology at one's own workplace by position in the hierarchy (in percentage)

a: leading   b: intermediate   c: office

worse   better

Direct system users were mostly office workers. However, it was only in central organisation (CA) that all office workers were directly involved; in the other places some groups of office workers were completely outside the new system. Persons in intermediate organisational positions were active direct system users in prison administration (PA) and elsewhere were just occasional users. Superiors were at most indirect users, that is they used services which entailed direct system use for their subordinates.

Most direct users put the learning time somewhere between two weeks and three months, whereas superiors tended to underestimate the time needed. Learning time was longest in CA where the system covered the information flow in the department as a whole. It was strikingly short in LOC/H where the future direct users had been in contact with the programmers during the period of programme development and had a terminal to work with while waiting for the system to be ready.

The level of mastery of system use varied from none at all to flexible use in several tasks, including uncommon tasks. Almost two out of three office workers and persons in intermediate positions mastered the system on the level of flexible use in common tasks, or alternatively, in simple routines, while the last third of them did not know how to use the system at all. More than half of the superiors either could not use the system or just knew about its possibilities and limitations, while some could perform simple tasks. Almost everybody emphasised individual motivation – positive attitudes and scrupulous attention to the tasks – as the main prerequisite for learning. Knowing the techniques and principles in computer science and system design was second on the list. After a year of experience with the system, workers felt that it was important to know the work well and to understand the information flow in the organisation.

The general pattern of expectations proved to be partially valid, when we examined actual experiences with the new technology by asking questions structured in the same way as those on expectations. Aspects where no change was expected really did remain stable: salary (98 per cent), organisational position (94 per cent), security of employment (90 per cent – some office workers were still worried) and appreciation of one's work (89 per cent). None of the expected positive consequences had been realised.

The quality of service to clients had improved (63 per cent), very noticeably in CA, although not quite as much as expected in other departments. Flexibility of organisational functioning did not improve as expected (only 47 per cent reported improvements) but remained at its former level. The discrepancy between the main appeal of advertisements on new information technology and actual experience was even wider: improvement in efficiency was reported only half as often as it was expected to take place (36 per cent). Fortunately, there were not many decreases in efficiency either.

The aspects which produced clear differences according to position showed interesting developments (see figure 2). The optimism so prevalent among superiors had largely evaporated, and the office workers found that expectations of improving their qualifications had partly been wishful thinking. On the other hand, fears about the impoverishment of work content had also proved to be exaggerated, and almost one-third of the office workers actually reported improvements. But their suspicions about the deterioration of working conditions and the social atmosphere of the workplace had been well founded. The group atmosphere had been especially vulnerable to the introduction of new information systems. The poor working conditions were not connected so much with ergonomic problems concerning the terminal as with the inappropriate location or insufficient number of terminals. These are problems which resulted from neglect of the needs of the direct users in the planning process.

Coping with technological changes

The aim of this study was to analyse how people act in changing situations, and specifically how office women integrate new technology into their work and how they cope with it. This involves not only adaptation to new working situations, but also to the ways people use to try to master the social situation in their work community. Previously, it was emphasised that in their social interactions, office workers produce and reproduce a work culture of their own. For this reason, different forms of qualitative methods were used when gathering research material in the offices investigated. The observations, interviews and discussions with groups and individuals focused on how office women coped at the level of their work community.[25]

Office workers in the prison administration office were distributed among the department sections in a decentralised way with one or two assigned to a functional unit of various specialists. The situation did not spontaneously lead to a common occupational identification of office workers. Other workers tended instead to see themselves as part of a group serving a common functional goal. Consequently, the coping strategies typical in the PA appeared to have a character of independence, sometimes bordering on isolation. With that in common, the coping strategies still ranged from enthusiasm to apprehension.

The information system in PA included a separate register which was delegated to two office workers. To begin with, there was only one terminal available for them, and since one of the office workers was also doing academic studies and was often absent, the other workers placed the terminal in her office. She felt a great challenge and became familiar with the system and adapted it to the current work. It was of primary importance to her that the information system be used efficiently as soon as possible since it would improve service to clients and make the work easier. She saw her own activeness as a counteraction to the computer professionals who did not know the concrete details involved in the register and were rather slow to understand her questions.

She used most of her free time for several weeks to prepare the system for use: she made manuals and took it upon herself to train other office workers. All this was done in addition to her normal work routines, without material rewards or relief from other duties. She actually saved the department significant training costs. As a result she enriched her own job – which was not her conscious aim – and at the same time, made herself indispensable. Such initiative was possible in PA, where the planning was relatively open-ended and allowed the users to be more active. However, while she was respected, she felt she could have used more emotional support. She was allowed great independence, was not controlled and was left alone – and consequently she felt lonely.

Other office workers in PA had a more contradictory attitude to the new information technology. Direct users felt apprehensive about the health risks of terminals, but at the same time they liked the technology. It made their work easier and produced a kind of "addiction". Typically each worker coped with the dilemma separately. The workplace culture in PA was quite permissive in that each office worker could choose between active involvement or quiet distancing. However, the differences in attitudes among the office workers created some emotional tensions, waivering between envy and trust.

The typical feature in the court of appeals was that group strategies developed.[26] This is understandable in the strictly hierarchical organisational context, which had already created the basis for distinct occupational categories and geographically united work groups of office workers. Among the registry office workers, this led to a common strategy of withdrawal, while the secretaries found a collective strategy of developing their individual work in the organisation.

The registry office workers appeared to be passive recipients of the new information system. They did not know much about it beforehand, and they did not try to influence the planning in any way. For them the introduction of the new system meant problems in social relationships and a change in the service to clients. One of the office workers in the registry was given the status of "main user" of the system. Her tasks and her contacts in the department widened, and the others began to think of her as the "mistress of secret knowledge". Decisions about work organisation which were made outside and above them thus created different statuses among the office workers. Formerly, they were a very integrated work community with common cultural orientations, acting together in their common responsibility for service to clients and actually controlling the information flow of the organisation. The new information system improved the service to clients, which was very important to the registry office workers. They could maintain a good image of the CA in outward contacts with the individual clients. At the same time, the quality of their social interaction was changing, because each worker had a separate task to perform.

The registry office workers criticised the introduction of the new information technology, which had taken place without their participation and without using their expertise in the actual handling of the information flow. The criticism and resistance took the form of complaints which remained within their own work group and discussions where they ridiculed the planners and belittled the importance of the changes. They believed that it would be useless to try to influence matters because of their place in the hierarchy. They just tried to hold on to their work community and to take care of the needs of clients.

The secretaries coped in a different way. They had not been in a work group, just a category in the occupational hierarchy of the CA, each inside her own room and engaged in her separate quota of cases. The new information system changed their situation in that routines increased in their work. Since there were not enough terminals for each of them, they had to wait, queue and take turns in using the system. This created opportunities to express their frustrations about the content and organisation of work and led eventually to the start of a common discussion group.

The secretaries were conscious of the importance of common action. They handled both the practical problems of their work and the organisational barriers which made their problems difficult to solve. But they went even farther; they analysed their own psychological adjustment to the hierarchy. They wanted to take the responsibility for improving the work and status of secretaries, which would have consequences on the total work organisation.

The coping strategies of the registry office workers were in many ways the opposite of the strategies of the secretaries. In the registry they wanted to *conserve* the former social community and maintain the common interpretation of their world. The secretaries, on the other hand, consciously set a goal of *change*. A process of differentiation was taking place in the registry, while the secretaries were becoming more integrated as a group. The strategy of the registry office workers was actually quite useful to the power structure of the hierarchy, while the strategy of the secretaries may lead to conflicts with the structure.

The two local courts were structurally quite alike, but the workplace culture differed decisively. LOC/T operated smoothly using standard hierarchical and bureaucratic methods, while LOC/H was like an extended family run by experienced office workers. LOC/T tried to follow as closely as possible the formal regulations about work and the division of tasks and to accept the new technology as something coming from the Ministry which should not be fussed about. Privately, the office workers were anxious and uncertain but had to live with their lack of information, and trust that nothing drastic would happen. Their strategy was one of adaptation and minimal change. They just waited for orders from superiors on how they should use the system, and used it as a mechanical tool to carry out their daily work as usual.

The office workers of LOC/H, even though they had no formal permission to participate in the planning process, started a discussion about it in the workplace. They believed that technological change should be taken seriously. Since the ISU needed their manual data base to build up the register, they took advantage of the regular contacts with programmers and made their own suggestions for making the system correspond better with the established practice of the office. Openness, curiosity and a desire to learn something new was typical in the LOC/H. Organisational ties to the trade union movement influenced both expectations and action. The office workers at LOC/H were also instrumental in setting up a committee to follow the social consequences of technological development in their union. The work culture of LOC/H allowed people to be active, and the office workers felt specially responsible for the social community of the workplace.

Coping strategies are either active or oriented to a more passive adjustment to the situation. The office women – or groups of office women – who used the active strategies either had jobs which gave them some autonomy or had positions which were somewhat higher within the category of the office workers (which in itself was low in the hierarchy). Passive adjustment strategies were typical in the lowest positions. Another important factor is also the general orientation to work: the active strategies seemed to demand an occupational identity, which was not well developed among the office workers who adopted passive strategies.

Conclusions and perspectives

Several conclusions can be drawn from this material. Clerical occupations are stabilising in number after a period of rapid growth. Women are the overwhelming majority in these occupations where tasks and status are differentiated by sex. Women are in the labour market to remain; what happens in the workplace is a serious matter to them. They are almost all organised in unions, and the unions have started to formulate their own policies concerning new technology. On the other hand, the employees' right to participate in the planning and control of the changes is controversial.

Political programmes are often not reflected in practices at the workplace. There are official decrees about the co-operation of different personnel groups in public administration, decrees which are scarcely known at the workplaces, let alone conscientiously followed. There are modern enterprises which give their employees a chance to participate in the introduction process, but this often occurs independently of political programmes or official pronouncements.

New information technology spreads in a society where it is encouraged ideologically and generally supported, even if it is accompanied by apprehensions.

The introduction of new information technology can today be characterised as determined by the market and introduced into the organisation through a hierarchical decision-making process. It is usually decided upon without any influence from the office women at the lower levels of the hierarchy, even though they will be affected most by its introduction.

New information technology has not created direct unemployment in clerical occupations. Organisations rely on the mechanism of natural attrition. The consequence is a structural problem for women outside the labour market, unless the prevailing trend of sex-segregation in education and occupational choice can be counteracted.

Degradation of work has not taken place as a consequence of the new technology. An overall picture of people working with new information technology shows people working under pressure and stress, but mostly with interesting and responsible tasks.

The invisible reality of much of women's office work provides a better understanding of the way work is changing. Women's office work produces and maintains social community and common frameworks of interpretation. Its interactional character and the need to maintain continuity require a special orientation which is provided by feminine socialisation. Many offices are not the "information factories" which are

215

the implicit models for formalising information flow into data systems. The visible routines are founded on a reality of essentially social character, where the female labour force is an unrecognised necessity.[27]

At present, the processes of technological change raise problems. Training is superficial and does not meet the requirements of the actual work – all the more so, when quite often there will be more work and faster work expected with less staff. The designers, the vendors, the decision-makers, as well as the users themselves, visualise the requirements, challenges and problems of the introduction of new technology as belonging to the individual and to be solved by the individual. The utility of this approach is supported by the need to fill the gap between superficial training and actual job requirements. But this approach does not resolve the underlying problem that the model for introduction ignores the social aspects of the work community and the way in which knowledge and traditional problem-solving methods are transmitted in an office. Discrepancies between theory and reality may vent themselves in the rupture of social relations at the workplace, of which there is already some evidence.

It is therefore important that research should point out these hidden processes to emphasise that the consequences of new information technology in office work are in reality consequences of the way organisations function and of how men and women act.

Notes

1 OECD Working Party on Information, Computer and Communications Policy: *Group of Experts on Economic Analysis of Information Activities and the Role of Electronics and Telecommunications Technologies*, Volume II, Background reports (Paris, 1980).

2 Central Statistical Office: *Position of women in Finland*, Statistical Surveys No. 72 (Helsinki, CSO, 1984).

3 M.-L. Anttalainen: *Naisten työt – miesten työt* [Women's jobs – men's jobs], Tasa-arvoasiain Neuvottelukunta, Valtioneuvoston kanslian julkaisuja 1980: 1 (Helsinki, Central Office of the Cabinet, 1980).

4 P. Korvajärvi; L. Rantalaiho: *Toimistoautomaatio ya Toimistotyö* [Office automation and office work], Tampereen yliopisto, Yhteiskuntatieteiden tutkimuslaitos [Research Reports of the Social Science Research Institute], sarja B 40/1984 (University of Tampere, 1984).

5 L. Rantalaiho: "Naiset toimistotyössä" [Women in office work], in L. Husu and M. Honkasal (ed.): *Työ, nainen ja tutkimus* [Work, women and research], VNK:n monisteita 1984:2 (Helsinki, Central Office of the Cabinet, 1984).

6 Työvoimatutkimus 1982, vuosihaastattelu [Labour Force Survey, Yearly Interview] Tilastotiedotus TY 1984:3, Tilastokeskus (Helsinki, CSO, 1984).

7   Central Statistical Office, op. cit.

8   E. Niinikoski and M. Kavonius: *Automaatioteemavuosi 1982-1983* [Theme year 1982-1983: Automation] (Helsinki, Suomen Teollisuustoimihenkilöiden Liitto STL (FFIE), 1983).

9   ibid.

10 Korvajärvi; Rantalaiho, op. cit.

11 T. Savaspuro: *Automaation ja atk:n kehityspuitteet kunnallishallinnossa* [The development frame of automation and EDP in municipal administration] Kunnallistaloudelliset opintopäivät Espoossa 12 August 1982 (Espoo, Conference on Municipal Economics, 1982).

12 *Teknologiakomitean mietintö* [Report of the Finnish Technology Committee] Komiteanmietintö 1980:55 (Helsinki, 1980).

13 Virkamiesliitto [Union of Civil Servants]: *Tietotekniikkaa ehdoillamme* [Information technology on our conditions], Rati-sarja n:03 (Helsinki, 1983).

14 Ministry of Social and Health Affairs: *Työntekijöiden osallistumismahdollisuuksia uuden teknologian suunnitteluun, kehittämiseen ja käyttöönottoon Käsittelevän sosiaali – ja terveysminis – teriöon työryhmän mietintö* [Report of a Special Commission of the Ministry of Social and Health Affairs on the Possibilities of Participation of Workers and Employees in the Planning, Development and Introduction of New Technology] (Helsinki, 1983).

15 *Automaatio kunnallishallinnossa* [Automation in municipal administration] (Helsinki, Kunnallisen alan rationalisointineuvottelukunta, 1981).

16 *Valtioneuvoston periaatepäätös rationalisointiyhteistyöstä valtion virastoissa* [Government recommendation on co-operation in administrative rationalisation in state administrative offices] 6 Nov. 1980 P 5623 (Helsinki, Valtion virkaehdot, 1983).

17 Central Statistical Office: *Työolotutkimus 1984: Työn haitat* [The quality of working life survey 1984: Working conditions] TY 1985:17 (Helsinki, CSO, 1985).

18 ibid.

19 TVK: Jäsentutkumus 1984 (Membership survey of the CSEF), Jyväskylä, 1984.

20 E.H. Wynn: *Office conversation as an information medium* (Berkeley, California, Department of Anthropology, University of California, 1979).

21 K. Sjörup and K. Thomsen: "Er teknologi magt?" [Is technology power?], in *Kvinder og teknologisk udvikling*, Konferenceindlaeg, Aalborg 21-23 Aug. 1985, 2nd Nordic Conference on Women, Science and Technology.

22 See, for example, H. Braverman: *Labor and monopoly capital* (New York, Monthly Review Press, 1974).

23 Korvajärvi and Rantalaiho: op. cit.; and P. Köonnilä: *Tietotekniikka ja toimistotyö* [Information technology and office work] Suomen Akatemian toimistoautomaatio-projektin tutkimuselosteita [Research Reports of the Office Automation Project, Social Science Council of the Finnish Academy] (Tampere, 1985).

24 H. Virtanen: *Toimistoautomaation käyttöönoton kynnyksellä* [On the threshold of office automation] Suomen Akatemian toimistoautomaationprojektin julkaisuja [Research Reports of the Office Automation Project, Social Science Council of the Finnish Academy], (Tampere, 1984).

25 B.-A. Sörensen: "Ansvarsrasjonalitet: om malmiddeltenkning blant kvinner" [Rationality of responsibility: On end-means thinking among women], in H. Holter

(ed.): *Kvinner i felleskap* [Women's collectives] (Oslo-Bergen-Tromsö, Universitetsforlaget, 1982; and I. Wagner: *Women in automated offices: Contradictory experiences – Individual and collective coping strategies*, Paper presented at IFIP Conference on Women, Work and Computerisation, Riva del Sole, 17-21 Sept. 1984.

26 E. Kallioniemi: *Työyhteisöön tuli toimistoautomaatio* [Computerised data system confronts the workplace community], Projektiraportti [Project Reports of the Social Science Research Institute] (Tampere, 1985).

27 A. Boman: *Omsorg och solidaritet – ohallbara argument?* [Caring and solidarity – untenable arguments?], Arbetsrapport 1983:1 (Stockholm, Arbetslivscentrum, 1983); and L. Rantalaiho: "Kvinnlig arbetsorientering och kontrosautomation" [Women's orientation to work and office automation], in *Sosiologia* 1/1985 (Helsinki), pp. 23-24.

218

8 New technologies in the service sector in Hungary

K. BALATON

The service sector in Hungary

General characteristics

Before the Second World War, Hungary was mainly an agricultural country. After 1945, Hungary started to build a socialist society, and has been a member State of the socialist countries' Council of Mutual Economic Assistance (CMEA) since 1949.

Along with the creation of state-owned enterprises and co-operatives, efforts were made to replace market conditions with central planning. In developing the economy, primacy was given to manufacturing, particularly to heavy industry. The role of the service sector was underestimated.

During the 1960s, it became obvious that underdevelopment of the service sector was undesirable, not only from the point of view of industrial production but also for the development of the economy as a whole. The role of services was re-evaluated, and greater emphasis was given to their development. The percentage of employees working in the service sector was 32.3 per cent in 1971; by 1981 it had risen to 38.6 per cent.

The retail sector.[1] The present structure of commercial activities is primarily the result of the radical changes introduced after 1945. Before then all trade was privately owned. By 1952 trading had become organised into state-owned and co-operative ownership. Organisational changes also resulted in rigid separation between industrial and commercial activities. Producing companies did not deal directly with consumers. Retail or trading companies were responsible for the distribution of goods produced.

Along with changes in the economic management system and the increasing role of the market, the function and structure of commercial activities also changed. The rigid separation between wholesale trade and retail trade diminished, and competition among trading organisations was allowed. Although state-owned and co-operative organisations have an overwhelming role, the number of private shops has increased. In 1982, 15,650 private shops operated in the retail sector, compared with 25,987 state-owned shops and 28,924 co-operatively owned shops.[2]

State-owned department stores (88 in 1982) are organised into the Centrum State Stores Company. Co-operative department stores (89 in 1982) belong to the Sk.la-Coop Association. Department stores have a mixed character. Typically, they sell clothing and appliances, but food departments are also becoming more and more frequent. In the food trade there are 22 regional companies, one nation-wide company (Csemege) and 12 companies in Budapest. Generally, one food-trading company and one or two retailing enterprises for appliances operate in each county. In Budapest, specialised companies for clothing and appliances are also found.

In 1971 domestic trade employed 8.3 per cent of all workers. This ratio has remained nearly unchanged. Sales turnover, on the other hand, has increased rapidly. In 1971 sales turnover in trading companies was 350,037 million Forints, and this value increased to 903,843 million forints in 1982.

Gross value of fixed assets applied in domestic trade rose from 24 billion forints to 71.1 billion forints between 1971 and 1982. The annual rate of increase was 6.9 per cent during those 11 years.

The banking sector.[3] In Hungary there is a so-called single-level banking system, which is also characteristic of other East European socialist countries. This means that banking policies are determined by the central bank, the National Bank of Hungary (NBH). There are some specialised banks but their banking policy is controlled by the NBH. Banks are mainly owned by the State, although some smaller financial institutions are owned by co-operatives.

Banks employ 20,000 people, 0.5 per cent of the employees in Hungary. The capital stock of the banks and financial institutions is about 10 billion forints, 0.5 per cent of the capital in Hungary.

The National Bank of Hungary (NBH) has a double role: it is a central bank and a credit or commercial bank. As the central bank of the country it has a monopoly on issuance of money, credit and money circulation and foreign exchange. It formulates the national credit policy and carries out parliamentary and governmental resolutions, especially on maintaining the approved ratio between credits and credit sources. The bank also collects and manages stocks in gold and foreign exchange. The bank has 7,000 employees. Aside from its central offices, it has 19 county head offices and 64 branches.

Besides the central bank, the State Development Bank (SDB) and the National Savings Bank (NSB) play a significant role. The first specialises in investment finance. The second accepts deposits and grants credits.

The Hungarian Foreign Trade Bank is a special bank for financial operations in connection with capitalist banks. It is a joint stock company with capital of 130,000 shares valued at 10,000 forints each. The bank grants loans mainly for investments which will improve the country's balance of foreign exchange in hard currency.

There are a few other specialised financial institutions. The Central Exchange and Credit Bank, a subsidiary of the National Bank of Hungary, specialises in financing innovative investments. It owns the Central Wechsel und Creditbank A.G. Niederlassung Wien in Austria. The Bankinghouse Centre collects debts from abroad in the name of Hungarian citizens and manages their property abroad and the income coming from that property. The Centre also manages the liquidation of firms.

The role of the banking system is increasing in the Hungarian economy. The structure of financial institutions will change as a result of banking reforms which have been started. The first steps towards a double-level banking system separating the functions of the issuing bank and that of the credit or commercial bank have been taken.

The health care system.[4] For the past three decades the basic aim in developing the health care system has been the gradual integration of the whole society into the social security system, making free medical service accessible to all. Preference has been given to the provision of out-patient services as the cheapest way to develop the public health sector.

The number of persons included in the system increased more than three times between 1945 and 1980 as the public health service expanded, and as the number of doctors increased from 10,000 to 30,000. During the same time the number of hospital beds increased from 40,000 to 97,000.

The network of public health institutions is based on a regional principle, so that every citizen has in principle the right to receive out-patient and in-patient service near his own home. In case of need for medical treatment, patients consult their regional panel doctor who will either care for them, send them to the regional special surgery, or if the doctor considers it necessary, send them to an appropriate hospital. In very serious cases he may send the patient to an institute offering specialised medical treatment. Out-patient and in-patient services are both divided into basic care and specialised care.

There are 4,200 basic service districts in the country. Each panel doctor is responsible for the care of 2,500 people on average. Specialised out-patient service is provided by the nearly 200 specialised clinics integrated with the general hospital nearest to them. Judicial and financial supervision of these institutions is provided by the city, metropolitan, district and county councils.

In-patient service is theoretically multi-levelled. Each general hospital is under council supervision; within this, the relatively smaller institutes are financed by the city councils or, in the case of the capital, by district councils. The larger hospitals belong directly to the county or municipal councils.

Fifty-three per cent of the council hospitals have fewer than 500 beds, while 27 per cent have more than 1,000 beds. The average number of beds is 630. When patients require special machines or instruments as well as higher professional knowledge, they fall within the sphere of the national institutes and university clinics. The 17 national institutes, the four university medical clinics and the Medical Post-graduate Institute are directly controlled by the Ministry of Health, which finances close to 20 per cent of the total beds.

Conditions of work in the service sector

One factor influencing working conditions in the service sector is the fact that there is full employment in Hungary, and in the service sector there is even a shortage of labour. This must be kept in mind when considering both the conditions of work and the introduction of new technology.

Conditions of work in Hungary are regulated by national-level directives for all sectors. The State sets salary and wage levels based on the kind of job. In the profit-making sectors, the actual level of earnings is dependent on the organisation's performance.

The economically active population consists of men between the ages of 14 and 60 and women between the ages of 14 and 55. Each employee is entitled to receive a pension upon retirement.

There is a five-day workweek, with Saturday and Sunday generally free. However, in the service sector it is frequently not possible to be free during the weekend, and in these cases a free day is provided on another day of the week.

The number of working hours per week is between 40 and 42. The 40-hour week is being introduced in more and more organisations. Part-time work is rare. Most employees work full-time; part-time work is mainly done by women with small children.

In the case of shift work, a financial incentive for the afternoon and night shifts is provided to fill the jobs.

Industrial relations

Trade unions in Hungary are organised by professional activity and follow the branch structure of the economy. There are, for example, trade unions of iron and metal industry workers, of chemical industry workers and of health-care workers. Trade unions on the national level are under the control of the Trade Unions National Council (SZOT). General trade union policy is decided by SZOT. Every trade union is composed of workplace units organised in enterprises and institutions. Only in the armed forces and police are there no trade unions.

In the workplace, most people belong to trade unions. Participation of workers in management of organisations is governed by national legislation. Participation in enterprise-level management may be direct and indirect. The possibility of giving opinions during workers' assemblies is a direct form of participation. Such assemblies are organised in connection with the most important decisions of an organisation, for example annual plan targets. Assemblies are held at enterprise and branch level.

The organisational structure of trade unions provides indirect ways of participating. At every workplace, trade union trustees are elected by the workers. These trustees are members of trade union councils at the organisation level, the approval of which is needed in most important decisions of the enterprises.

There is a question as to how worker participation functions in practice. The development of democratic styles is a current question, and many central-level organisations have dealt with it in the last few years. Tradition and overcentralisation of the political and economic sphere have not encouraged the development of workplace democracy. Currently, the political programme of the ruling Hungarian Socialist Workers' Party emphasises the need for developing democracy.

Representatives of trade unions participate in final decision-making on the introduction of new technology, but it is difficult to evaluate the actual extent of their influence.

New technologies in the service sector

Introduction of new technology

Introduction of microelectronics in Hungary started relatively recently. Until the end of the 1960s only a few companies used electronic data processing. Then, in 1969 the East European socialist countries decided on a joint programme for the production and distribution of computers. As a result of this decision, Hungary introduced a programme in 1971 to expand the use of computers in business enterprises. The ministries supervising enterprises became responsible for the application of computers. They provided financial support to companies introducing computers, with a strong preference for computers produced in the East European countries.

The ministries created branch-level and regional computer centres for meeting the data-processing needs of enterprises and institutions. In many cases, it was necessary to force companies to use the capacity of the computers installed.

Until the middle of the 1970s, central initiatives continued to be the primary moving force in computerisation.[5] Business enterprises went along with the government programme in order to maintain good relationships with the supervising ministries. The result was a generally low level of application. It was only important to *use* microelectronics, not to use them effectively. From an economic point of view, these applications were not justifiable.

This type of development process may seem surprising in the light of the large number of empirical studies in Western countries which prove the competitive advantages of using microelectronics. However, in the Hungarian economy, though large-scale organisations play an overwhelming role, competition between organisations usually does not exist. Consequently, companies are not forced by competition to introduce more highly developed methods in manufacturing goods and providing services.

More sophisticated applications were also restricted by technical problems. There are often complaints about the reliable functioning of computers produced in East European countries. Another technological factor is the underdevelopment of the communications system in Hungary, which frequently makes it impossible to introduce remote data processing.[6] From the end of the 1970s certain signs of change began to emerge. Instead of central initiatives, the real needs of enterprises became more important. Changes in the economic management system encouraged greater independence of organisations and an increasing role for competition in the economy. An increase in exports is a primary aim of economic policy, and enterprises have to use microelectronics to be able to compete in the world market.

Main types of advanced technology in the service sector

The use of advanced technology in retailing, banking and health care started with electronic data processing (EDP). The introduction of EDP systems became widespread during the 1970s. The national computer programme established in 1971 played a decisive role in the spread of EDP. During the first period, up to 1975, computers were mainly used for accounting purposes and were not linked to the basic functions of service organisations. Data-processing systems of this period were mainly off-line and provided only limited possibilities for direct use at the managerial level. Another characteristic of early EDP applications was the low level of integration of the different functions of organisations. Disadvantages of these early systems, including the relatively high cost of data processing, soon became obvious.

The second phase of computer applications has been characterised by an increased level of integration. Specifically, this has entailed integrated management information systems, and on-line systems to provide up-to-date information for decision-making.

Advanced technologies in retailing. EDP applications, such as daily registration of sales turnover and changes in stock levels, are used more and more frequently in the retail sector. This information is used in re-ordering decisions, making possible an increased level of service activity. More advanced uses of new technology are also emerging. Some point-of-sale terminals and visual display units have been installed to register or record sales turnover. Both systems provide the possibility of getting up-to-date information on sales and stock levels at any time necessary.

Department stores using point-of-sale terminals are either self-service stores selling items from shelves, or department stores which make sales based on displays of samples. In the first type of store, only the cashiers and not the shop assistants are in direct contact with an automated system.

Shop assistants in department stores making sales based on display samples do work directly with the computerised system. Sample items are shown in the store, but purchased items are delivered to the customer's home from the warehouse. Shop assistants give information on product characteristics, stock levels and shipment dates by using the display terminals placed in the showrooms. They then use the terminals to make reservations or orders for buyers. Shop assistants use product catalogues to know the identification code numbers of the goods. After making the order, they fill in the "buyer's card" manually. The buyer then pays for the goods at the cashier's desk.

Shop assistants have to have the qualification of a commercially skilled worker to obtain their jobs, but this is unrelated to use of the new technology. Using the display terminals is relatively easy to learn. Sales assistants were taught by computer technicians how to use the new systems at the time they were introduced. Newly hired workers learn how to work with terminals from their colleagues. The mode of use is either data entry (making reservations or orders) or retrieval (of stock information). No dialogue mode of use is applied.

Sales assistants having work experience with new technologies theoretically have an advantage over those who work with traditional methods. However, the labour shortage in the shop assistant occupation eliminates this advantage. Furthermore, the equipment is easy to learn and to use.

Shop assistants interviewed were satisfied with the new technology. After the installation of new equipment, certain signs of stress were observed, but after a few months they disappeared. Without the new technology to perform the same task volume, more shop assistants would be required. Considering the shortage of labour, greater use of new technologies is foreseen.

The introduction of new technology occurred at the same time as the opening of new department stores in each case. Since then the technologies have not changed.

Another retail occupation affected by the new technology is that of cashier. Two types of electronic point-of-sale system may be found in Hungary. The most developed application is represented by laser scanning. Use of this technology is limited by the lack of general use of European article numbering system (EAN) codes by producers. It is anticipated that consumer goods will be supplied with EAN codes in the future. Retail units currently using laser scanning have to supply items with codes in their storerooms.

In less-developed applications, cashiers have to key in item codes for automatic registration of sales. This solution is used in the system where sales are based on samples.

The cashiers register sales, totalling up the value of sales by using the terminal. The mode of use is data entry, except for information retrieval to get total sales value.

There is no need for professional qualifications to be a cashier. Most of the cashiers have secondary-school education. Commercially skilled workers may also be found in these jobs. To be promoted from cashier to shop assistant requires the qualification of a commercially skilled worker. However, in both positions, educational background is unrelated to use of the new technology, since learning to work with point-of-sale terminals is quite easy and takes only a few days. Likewise, there is no direct connection between the use of new technology and salary levels.

The basic salary of cashiers is determined by national standards and the general profitability of organisations. There is also a second salary element dependent on sales turnover. The turnover-dependent salary may represent as much as 40 per cent of earnings. There is no direct connection between the use of new technology and salary levels.

Cashiers expressed both positive and negative reactions to the new technology. Typical reactions were the following:

- the new system is faster than the old one;
- after learning the system it is easier to use;
- the workload has decreased;
- there are better possibilities of having more interesting jobs.

The most frequent negative reactions were as follows:

- more attention and accuracy is needed;
- the work is monotonous;
- the equipment is unreliable;
- communications with colleagues are more limited.

Advanced technologies in banking. In banking, EDP systems are generally used for monitoring credit and cash turnover and for making financial analyses and statistics. Back-office and front-office terminals have been put into use. In 1982, Hungary joined the SWIFT (Society for World-wide Interbank Financial Telecommunications) system, so terminals are used to send and receive information on financial transactions.

In the Hungarian banking system, terminals are used most extensively for foreign exchange operations with the SWIFT system. Of particular interest, therefore, are the dealers, employees whose responsibility it is to carry out cash and credit transactions. Dealers have direct contact with a number of banks of the world. By using microelectronic devices, they have day-to-day information on exchange and interest rates. Their tasks include raising and repaying short-term and medium-term loans and extending credit. Computer print-outs on repayment terms provide basic information for their work.

Dealers work continuously with microelectronic equipment. Reuter monitors are on all day, and the dealing system is used more and more frequently in making contracts. The mode of use of terminals is dialogue: messages are received and sent out to partner banks.

A transaction may be started either on initiation of the dealer, or by request of the partner bank. Each dealer has a workstation from which the electronic devices can be put into operation. Approximately half of the transactions are settled by phone, the other half by the Reuter dealing system. The transactor may decide autonomously on purchase, sale or credit transactions, except in the case of the raising of medium-term credit. The application of microelectronics in this function started in 1975. Since that time the technology has changed three times. Old equipment has been replaced by more sophisticated equipment.

The qualifications demanded of dealers are quite high. A university-level degree in economics is required, as well as fluency in at least one of the world languages. Promotional opportunities within the bank are likewise high. To be a successful dealer requires frequently updating one's professional knowledge. Dealers participate in study tours abroad, ranging from one day to three months, to expand their knowledge of the trade.

Salaries are based on wage rates which set lower and upper limits to salaries, depending on the job, education and years worked. Salaries do not depend on actual performance and work productivity, but differences in efficiency are taken into account when bonuses are allocated.

The working hours are 7.30 a.m. to 4.00 p.m., but overtime is very often needed. The number of staff is not keeping pace with the growing business turnover. The amount of work depends on the fluctuation of exchange rates. When they change, business turnover is higher and the workload increases.

Dealers have positive opinions on the help of microelectronics in their jobs. Without the equipment, business turnover would be much less. Some of them expressed a need for newer generations of microelectronics.

Advanced technology in health care. Microelectronics-based automatic analysers are used in the laboratories of some hospitals. The present phase of development aims to connect these analysers to hospital-wide computer systems.

The work of laboratory assistants follows a regular routine. Their daily work starts with calibration of the equipment. Samples to be analysed arrive from the wards during the morning. The assistants manually register each sample, then fill up the equipment with the samples. The analysers automatically make the different measurements and provide the results, which the assistants record manually. Results are collected and sent back to the wards in the afternoon. The assistants finish their work by cleaning the equipment.

The daily hours of the assistants are from 7.30 a.m. to 4.15 p.m., with one assistant on duty at all times to meet urgent requests from the wards.

Laboratory assistants have secondary-school education in chemical sciences. Besides possessing professional knowledge, they have to learn to work with the new equipment. Unfortunately, career possibilities are rather limited, and the salary is a moderate to low one. Consequently there is a shortage of laboratory assistants in hospitals.

Laboratory assistants who work with the new technology are generally pleased with the higher level of productivity and increased reliability of automatic analysers.[7] The automatic analysers have been in place for ten years, with more and more sophisticated equipment being put into operation.

Overall impact of new technology on jobs

The influence of microelectronics can be analysed according to the following dimensions: specialisation, routinisation, discretion, required skills and career prospects.

Specialisation of jobs may be analysed by looking at the number of tasks to be performed in a certain job. As a consequence of the introduction of microelectronics, rather specialised new jobs have emerged. Data-entry jobs are a good example, where the entire job consists of one type of activity.

The introduction of microelectronics is sometimes carried out with a new division of labour within the function influenced. In order to shorten the necessary learning time, a few employees specialise in tasks closely connected with the new system, while others continue to perform their traditional tasks. The first group of employees experience an increase in specialisation while the others are unaffected.

A third type of change in specialisation may be observed when the operation of the new devices increases the content of existing jobs. Specialisation is decreased and variability within jobs increased, especially when monotonous clerical tasks are replaced by automated data processing.

Routinisation is measured by the frequency of performing tasks within a certain job. Routinisation is closely connected to the level of specialisation. Increased specialisation results in rather routinised jobs. Routinisation is generally increased in jobs related to data registration and input.

Discretion of jobholders was analysed according to the following characteristics: decisions on time to be allocated to perform tasks; physical location and movement; use of equipment in performing tasks; decisions on specific tasks within the job; and decisions on information to be used.

According to the above measures, discretion is more restricted in jobs directly connected to the new technology. Within the job the introduction of microelectronics results in decreased autonomy. Pre-programmed equipment generally determines the sequence of tasks and time available. Working with the machinery reduces the employees' possibilities of deciding on physical location and movement.

The skills necessary to perform tasks have shown different tendencies. One type of change is the necessity of increased skills in order to be able to operate the equipment. Old skills may become unnecessary. For example, automated diagnosis replaces traditional analytic methods. There is also a tendency towards a decrease in skills used. With the technological development of microelectronics, programming and handling of equipment has become easier, and their operation does not require highly skilled employees.

Concerning career possibilities we have not found meaningful changes within the organisation. Prospects depend on other factors than the new technology. There is a new tendency, however, in interorganisational career prospects. Those who have the theoretical knowledge and empirical experience are often offered jobs with organisations starting to adopt microelectronics. Middle-level managers in the field of operating new technology in newly innovating organisations are mainly recruited from firms having experience in working with microelectronics.

Technological and organisational design options

Characteristics of decisions to introduce new technology

Where new technology was introduced at the same time as a new organisation, or a new division within an organisation, was created, there seemed to be a definite intention to create an up-to-date information system in the new units. Cost-benefit analyses showed investment in new technology to be profitable. Practical reasons existed which were even more important. In retailing, for example, lack of storage capacity and the great distance from the warehouse made it necessary to introduce a fast and reliable information system. Managerial sensitivity toward new technology solutions also counted as an important factor.

Where technological developments were introduced into existing settings, there were many factors contributing to the decision to adopt microelectronics. Pressures for increased volume together with labour shortages, particularly in the service sector, have directed attention toward new technology with higher productivity. The need for greater

230

speed in performing tasks – faster laboratory analyses, banking services provided in less time, more rapid and reliable information on stock levels – has also led to the use of microelectronics.

Economic rationalisation of investment played only a limited role. This is partly because it is difficult to appraise the economic benefits of a sophisticated information system. Cost-benefit analyses, however, did have a significant role in certain cases. We analysed cases where organisations changed from using the computers of other enterprises to establishing their own computer centre. The increasingly high cost of subcontracting work and the lack of up-to-date information led organisations to introduce their own computer system. The necessity of replacing old electromechanical devices also created a favourable condition for the introduction of microelectronics.

Another factor in the introduction of new technologies is the professional ambition of decision-makers, or of the specialists advising them, and their preference for more sophisticated solutions. Highly qualified professionals who are extremely enthusiastic about microelectronics can be found in every organisation using the new technology. In certain cases, mainly in hospitals, the application of microelectronics was connected to scientific research. A desire to be a pioneer within the sector also influenced the introduction of new technologies.

The foregoing were internal factors. To get a full picture it is necessary to look also at external influences. After the government's computerisation programme was introduced in 1971, ministries became responsible for initiating broad-scale computer applications. Some organisations were regarded as model units within the sector. This occurred when ministry-level initiatives meshed with managerial con- cepts. Introduction of new technologies was then realised as a joint effort. In one case, specialists appointed by the ministry were directly involved in designing computer applications. In another case, the general manager of the organisation was at the same time the head of a computer application unit within the ministry.

Another outside factor can be found in the relationship between manufacturers and users of microelectronic equipment. In one of the cases reviewed, the user organisation had a contract with a manufacturer for testing new equipment. This provided mutual benefits. New equipment reached the user as soon as new products were developed. Successful testing then resulted in orders for new equipment.

The spread of microelectronics was promoted by the positive experiences of some organisations. In some cases top managers of organisations participated in study tours which affected their decisions to introduce new technology.

Among the factors influencing decision-making, we have to mention financial issues. Even though prices of microelectronic equipment are radically decreasing in world markets, East European prices are kept rather high. The joint production and distribution programme of these countries also covers the co-ordination of price levels.[8] The high cost of equipment deters the wider use of microelectronics.

The decision process is rather complicated when the users prefer to purchase microelectronics produced in Western countries. Besides having to have the development funds in Hungarian currency, companies have to obtain the authorisation for converting the currency. The ministries are also involved in the decision.

At first it may seem surprising that the cost of using the new technology was only a minor factor for both profit and non-profit organisations. However, in profit-making organisations, it is possible to build costs into the price of services; in the case of non-profit organisations, increased costs are covered by the budget. Sensitivity to cost level is relatively low not only in Hungary but also in other socialist countries.

Outside factors have affected operating costs, but until 1985, operating costs were not an important factor in arriving at decisions. Under the economic regulation system introduced in 1985, cost levels have become much more important in calculations and may restrict economically unjustifiable applications, for example batch-type data processing for accounting purposes.

Who are the decision-makers?

The decision process may be better understood if we look at who the initiators of innovation are. When looking at the whole process of decision-making, the persons really involved are the top-level managers, the heads of organisational and/or computer departments and the heads of functional departments who use the new technology in their daily work.

Top-level managers play an active role in the introduction of new technologies for two reasons. First, the innovation is usually an issue of strategic importance for the organisation. Second, outside influences, particularly from upper levels of the ministry, are brought to bear on those at the top level in the organisation.

Another group of initiators are the middle-level managers and highly skilled professionals. The professionnals have knowledge of possible applications of new technology and are sensitive to the most recent solutions. They often work in administrative or computer departments.

The decision-making process generally involved approval of the initial design, followed by a detailed plan for installation and introduction, discussed and approved by top-level managers. Representatives of trade unions participate in final decision-making, but their influencing power could not be observed in even one case. Employees affected by the new technology were generally informed only after the decision on introduction was made.

Changes in organisational structure due to the introduction of new technology

Only limited changes may be observed in organisational structures. The most obvious change is the creation of a new unit under the control of top-level managers.

A more meaningful change is the emergence of a new, professional type of hierarchy which exercises control over activities affected by the new technology. It has often been predicted that control would be more centralised with the application of microelectronics. In the cases we reviewed the locus of decision-making has hardly changed. There is in fact a possibility of centralisation of control, but top managers have not opted to use the new technology in that way. Their perceptions about the necessary level of centralisation have a direct influence on the outcome. One of the directors interviewed, for example, said: "I am aware of the increased possibility of direct control, but I think it is not my task to control day-to-day processes at lower levels".

There is a tendency toward increased formalisation as a result of the new technology. Procedures have to be adjusted to the standardised functioning of equipment. In addition to its direct impacts on specific functions, increased formalisation may be observed in functions connected to them through the information-processing network.

Influence of new technology on organisational processes

To analyse changes in organisational processes due to the introduction of new technology, the discussion below is divided into two categories: physical processes, and data processing and information flow.

In some cases, the application of new technology was not directly connected to a physical process, for example data processing for accounting purposes. In other cases, technology had a close connection with basic processes, such as laboratory analysis, flow of goods in department stores, and so on.

No basic changes have been observed regarding the physical processes. The main phases and their sequence remained the same. Smaller changes, however, did occur, such as increased speed, decreased number of interruptions and more integration of processes.

Information flow connected to physical processes changed radically. The volume of manually performed tasks decreased, according to the level of automation. Tasks to be performed changed, as did procedures and techniques used. The whole process became much more standardised.

Degrees of change in processes depended on the level of automation. From this point of view the following questions merit further investigation:

- to what degree is it necessary to maintain manual intervention;
- are there possibilities for decision-making interventions during the execution of processes;
- does information processing directly follow physical processes or is it performed after a time lag?

The more sophisticated the equipment used, the more changes in processes may be observed.

In decision-making, the use of microelectronics changes the type, form and frequency of information used. Routine-type decisions are partly made by the technological system. With these changes in decision-making, quality control reached a higher level than before.

Overview

The application of new technologies involves changes in both occupations and organisational structures. The extent of these changes varies according to the level of increase in the automatic execution of tasks. When only a limited number of functions is involved and microelectronics are used at a low level of systems integration, changes may be observed only on an individual job level. From the employees' point of view, the consequences are increased control by machines and limited possibilities for social contact with colleagues. As the new technology extends to more and more functions of organisations, and as highly automated integrated systems are used, the changes also become obvious in organisational structures. Our findings support N.M. Carter's conclusion: "As the extent of computer utilisation increases, the division

234

of labour as reflected by functional diversification, functional specialisation, and functional differentiation will also increase".[9]

Certain questions need to be answered concerning the effects of new technologies. One of these questions is whether the consequences for employment and for organisational structure are predetermined outcomes or are variables which may be influenced. According to our experience, we may state that, in general, consequences are not automatic and that specific outcomes may be influenced.

There is a long-standing debate on the connection between the introduction of computers and centralisation of control. Many authors argue that computerisation will result in increased centralisation.[10] From our experience we conclude that integrated systems using microelectronic technology provide possibilities for increased centralisation of control but the actual outcome is dependent on the intentions of the decision-makers. The technical sophistication of up-to-date systems may, however, also provide the possibility of decentralised control. Political considerations behind the introduction of microelectronics are important factors in understanding the consequences.

Power relationships within organisations cannot be overlooked. In highly professional organisations such as hospitals, doctors influenced the introduction of the new technologies. That situation did not exist in retailing and banking. In certain cases, pressure against organisational changes proved to be so strong that they prevented the successful implementation of new technology. Reluctance to change was observable, especially when the number and content of jobs belonging to certain departments or units had to be changed. The necessity of organisational changes for successful implementation is supported by the available literature. Vollmann et al., for example, conclude: "Many successful implementors now see that the key is to change the organisation to match the system, rather than vice versa".[11]

Another important question is the influence of new technology on the quality of working life. One of the extreme viewpoints is that computers and automation result in routinised jobs and, in this way, create boring workp leading to alienation.[12] Negative consequences are not inevitable. A crucial factor seems to be whether employees are involved in designing the workplace and working conditions. If they are not, fewer chances exist for avoiding negative consequences. No cases were observed where employees at a lower hierarchical level were involved in the design phase.

In Western countries, a debate is going on as to whether new technologies will increase employment or not. In Hungary and other socialist countries, the situation is quite different. Here the problem is not one of creating full employment but solving the problem of "effective" employment. This is especially true of the service sector where there is a shortage of labour. Higher productivity realised by the application of new technologies may help to solve this problem and to improve the quality of services.

Notes

1   This section is based on G. Kiss: *A magyar beikereskedelem általános jellemzöi* [General characteristics of the Hungarian domestic trade], Research paper (1984).

2   Central Statistical Office: *Yearbook of Domestic Trade* (Budapest, 1982).

3   This section is based on Zs. Járai: *A magyar bankrendszer rövid leirása* [Short description of the Hungarian banking system], Research paper (1984).

4   This section is based on A. László: *A magyar egészségügyi ellátás müködési mechanizmusa* [The operational mechanism of the Hungarian health provision system], Research paper (1985).

5   P. Tam.s: "A számitástechnika társadalmi környezetének jellemzöiröl" [About the characteristics of social environment of computerisation], in *Társadalomkutatás* [Social Research], 1983, No.1.

6   T. Vámos: *Hazánk és a müszaki haladás* [Hungary and technological development] (Budapest, Magvetö, 1984).

7   I. Branyiczki: *A Szekszárdi Kórház esete* [The case of the Szeksz.rd Hospital], Research paper (1984).

8   F. Nyitrai: "A számitástechnika alkalmazása hazánkban, a fejlödés fö irányai" [Application of computers in our country, the main directions of development], in *Vezetés-szervezés* [Management-organisation], 1984, No. 12.

9   N.M. Carter: "Computerization as a predominant technology: Its influence on the structure of newspaper organizations", in *Academy of Management Journal*, 1984, Vol. 27, No. 2.

10 For example, see T.L. Whisler: *The impact of computers on organization* (New York, Praeger, 1970).

11 T.E. Vollmann, W.L. Berry and D.C. Whyback: *Manufacturing planning and control systems* (Homewood, Illinois, Irwin, 1984).

12 H.A. Simon: *The new science of management decision* (Englewood Cliffs, New Jersey, Prentice Hall, 1977).

Index

credit institutions *see* banking
customers and clients, relations with, 3, 19-20
  in Finland, 208, 210, 212, 213
  in Germany, 19-20, 173, 178-9, 180-1, 184
  in Japan, 138, 147
  in Norway, 20, 39-41, 50, 55
  in United Kingdom, 97, 103, 104, 107
data capture units, 116, 118, 123
data processing industry, Japanese, 16, 133, 161-8, 169
decision-making *see* choice of technology
deskilling *see* skill requirements
dialogue systems, 12, 54-61, 71

EFT (electronic funds transfer), 5, 138
  at the point of sale (EFT/POS), 96, 99, 102, 104, 107, 118-19
EPOS (electronic point-of-sale) terminals 5, 9, 11, 14, 15, 16, 112-13
  and electronic funds transfer, 96, 99, 102, 104, 107, 118-19
  in Hungary, 14, 226-7
  in Japan, 9, 11, 15, 133, 143-51
  in Norway, 15
  in United Kingdom, 5, 16, 112-16, 119-25
European Article Numbering (EAN) system 5, 113, 175, 226

facsimile machines, 129, 133, 154
financial services *see* banking
Finland, 13, 16, 17, 18, 19, 21-2, 189-216
France, retail trade in, 118
future development of office work, 73-5

Germany, Federal Republic of, 7, 8, 11-12, 18, 19-20, 171-86
  banking services, 6-7, 13, 93, 171, 173, 176-81, 182-6

insurance companies, 13, 171, 173, 176-9, 181-6
retail and wholesale trade, 6, 113, 171, 172, 173, 174-6, 182-6
Government administration
  in Finland, 190, 192, 193, 195, 196, 201, 203-14, 215
  in Germany, 171, 173
  in Japan, 151-61, 169
Griffiths Report (1983) (United Kingdom), 80, 84

health services, 5-6, 12, 17-18
  in Hungary, 221-2, 223, 225, 228-9, 231, 234, 235
  in United Kingdom, 6, 9, 13, 79, 80-92, 125-6
Hedberg, B., 107
hierarchy *see* organisational structure
home
  banking, 102, 107, 118
  shopping, 116, 118, 150
  working, 75, 196
Hungary, 6, 8, 9, 21, 219-36
  banking services, 13-14, 220-1, 225, 227-8, 231, 235
  health services, 221-2, 223, 225, 228-9, 231, 234, 235
  retail trade, 219-20, 225-7, 230, 234, 235

Illich, I., 82
insurance companies, 1, 11
  in Finland, 191, 192, 196, 201
  in Germany, 13, 171, 173, 176-9, 181-6
  in Switzerland, 56-61
intensive care units, 5, 6, 12, 90-1
Italy, retail trade in, 113

Japan, 4, 8, 11, 12, 18
  banking services, 6, 7-8, 13, 17, 133, 135-43
  data-processing industry, 16, 133, 161-8, 169
  local government, 151-61, 169

Shimada, T., 134
skill requirements, 2, 3, 10, 12-15
  in Finland, 13, 191, 195-6, 197, 207,
    208, 211
  future developments, 74
  in Germany, 13, 178, 179, 180,
    182-5, 186
  in Hungary, 13-14, 226, 228, 230
  in Japan, 15, 133-4
    banking services, 13, 138-40
    data-processing industry, 164,
      165-6
    local government, 158-9
    retail and wholesale trade, 147-8,
      149
  in Norway, 14, 15, 29, 31-2, 36-9, 42,
    50
  in Switzerland, 62, 68
  in United Kingdom, 14, 77
    banking services, 13-14, 94, 100,
      101-2, 104, 106, 107, 126
    health service, 13, 88-9, 126
    retail trade, 14, 15, 124, 126
social relationships *see* communication
socio-technical systems design, 22-3,
  54, 73
software development, 12, 13, 54-61,
  71, 161-8
stress *see* pressure of work
structure *see* organisational structure
Sweden, 39, 191, 194
  banking services, 93, 107
SWIFT (Society for World-wide Inter-
  bank Financial Telecommunications), 227
Switzerland, 17, 53-75
  choice of technology, 12, 20-1, 22,
    53, 54-61, 72-3
  organisational structure, 9, 10, 61-73

Taylorist-style restructuring, 10, 201
technological choice *see* choice and
  introduction of technology
temporary office workers, Finnish, 197
tension *see* pressure of work

trade unions
  in Finland, 192, 193-5, 196, 204, 205,
    214, 215
  in Hungary, 223, 233
  in Japan, 130-1
    banking services, 137, 142
    data-processing industry, 162-3,
      166, 168
    local government, 155-7, 160
    retail and wholesale trade, 146-7,
      150
  in Norway, 26-8, 42, 44-7, 50-1
  in United Kingdom, 79, 126
    banking services, 79, 94, 96, 97,
      98, 106
    health service, 79, 80, 85-6
    retail trade, 79, 109, 110, 119-20,
      121, 124, 126
training, 15, 16
  in Finland, 191, 197, 199, 201-2, 207,
    216
  in Hungary, 226-7, 228-9
  in Japan, 15, 131, 148
  in Norway, 15, 32, 36, 37, 40, 47-9, 51
  in United Kingdom, 16, 89, 102,
    119-20
truncation, 96, 99, 102, 107

unions *see* trade unions
United Kingdom, 9, 11, 14, 77-126
  banking services, 11, 12, 16, 79-80,
    93-107, 125-6
  choice of technology, 21, 94,
    95-100, 106
  organisational structure, 7-8, 9,
    94, 102-7, 125
  health service, 6, 9, 13, 79, 80-92,
    125-6
  retail trade, 5, 9, 15, 16, 79-80,
    107-26
United States
  banking services, 93
  health services, 90
  retail trade, 5, 112, 113, 116, 118

Vollmann, T.E., 235

306 · 36